PNEUMOCYSTIS CARINII PNEUMONIA

LUNG BIOLOGY IN HEALTH AND DISEASE

Executive Editor: **Claude Lenfant**

Director, National Heart, Lung, and Blood Institute
National Institutes of Health
Bethesda, Maryland

PNEUMOCYSTIS CARINII PNEUMONIA

PATHOGENESIS • DIAGNOSIS • TREATMENT

Edited by

Lowell S. Young

University of California at Los Angeles
Center for the Health Sciences
Los Angeles, California

MARCEL DEKKER, INC.   New York • Basel

Library of Congress Cataloging in Publication Data

Main entry under title:

Pneumocystis carinii pneumonia.

    (Lung biology in health and disease ; v. 22)
    Includes bibliographies and indexes.
    1. Interstitial plasma cell pneumonia.
2. Pneumocystis carinii. I. Young, Lowell S.
II. Series. [DNLM: 1. Pneumonia, Interstitial
Plasma Cell. W1 LU62 v.22 / WC 209 P738]
RC772.I56P58 1984   616.2'41   84-14280
ISBN 0-8247-7077-3

Marcel Dekker, Inc.
270 Madison Avenue, New York, New York 10016

Current printing (last digit):
10 9 8 7 6 5 4 3 2 1

Printed in the United States of America

CONTRIBUTORS

Marilyn S. Bartlett, M.S. Associate Professor, School of Medicine/Allied Health, Indiana University School of Medicine, Indianapolis, Indiana

Michael S. Gottlieb, M.D. Assistant Professor, Division of Clinical Immunology-Allergy, Department of Medicine, University of California School of Medicine, Los Angeles, California

Jerome Groopman, M.D.* Assistant Professor, Division of Hematology-Oncology, Department of Medicine, University of California School of Medicine, Los Angeles, California

Beryl Jameson, M.B., Ch.B., F.R.C.Path. Consultant Microbiologist, Department of Microbiology, Royal Marsden Hospitals, London, England

Henry Masur, M.D. Deputy Chief, Critical Care, Medicine Department, Clinical Center, National Institutes of Health, Bethesda, Maryland

James W. Smith, M.D. Professor, Department of Pathology, Indiana University School of Medicine, Indianapolis, Indiana

Peter D. Walzer, M.D.† Staff Physician, Infectious Disease Section, Lexington Veterans Administration Medical Center, and Associate Professor, Department of Medicine, University of Kentucky College of Medicine, Lexington, Kentucky

---

Present affiliations:
*Assistant Professor, Division of Hematology-Oncology, Department of Medicine, Harvard University School of Medicine, and Attending Physician, New England Deaconess Hospital, Boston, Massachusetts
†Co-Chief, Infectious Disease Section, Cincinnati Veterans Administration Medical Center, and Associate Professor, University of Cincinnati School of Medicine, Cincinnati, Ohio

Lowell S. Young, M.D. Professor, Division of Infectious Diseases, Department of Medicine, University of California at Los Angeles, Center for the Health Sciences, Los Angeles, California

Phillip C. Zakowski, M.D. Lecturer, Division of Infectious Diseases, Department of Medicine, University of California School of Medicine, Los Angeles, California

FOREWORD

Most of us who are asked to name how the great advances in modern
medicine and surgery have come about, would probably respond by listing
some Nobel laureates and the discoveries closely linked with their names:
for example, Roentgen and X-rays; Koch and the tubercle bacillus; Fleming
and penicillin; Enders and culture of polio virus; Banting and insulin. Yet,
once in awhile, an event that is ineligible for a Nobel Prize has had just as
important an impact on medical advance as one that was eligible and won
an award. One such event was Abraham Flexner's 1910 report "Medical
Education in the United States and Canada" that resulted in a considerable
decrease in the number of American medical schools and a considerable
increase in their quality and in the scientific content of their curricula.
Another was the opening of the Johns Hopkins Medical School in 1893,
staffed by four professors, each outstanding as a scientist in his specialty
and each believing in joining scientific research, medical education, and
patient care.

Sometimes a book or a series of books has had a strong influence on
the advance of medical science. One such book was the first edition of
Osler's *Medicine* (1892) because Osler's emphasis on how little physicians
knew for sure led John Rockefeller's adviser on philanthropy to recommend the building of the great Institute for Medical Research, which
opened in 1904 and for decades was the foremost institution for research
in basic medical sciences in the United States. Another was the first
(1941) edition of Goodman and Gilman's *Pharmacological Basis for
Medical Practice* that revolutionized teaching and research on the action
and use of drugs; as one professor of pharmacology stated in 1941, no
professional pharmacologist could from then on teach at a lower level
than that of the superb text used by his students!

In the field of respiration and the lungs, there are some classic
monographs and a comprehensive *Handbook of Physiology* that have

v

heightened the interest of scientists, students, and physicians in this subject and stimulated them to enter pulmonary research. One can safely predict that this new series of monographs, "Lung Biology in Health and Disease," will have an even greater impact on young (and older) researchers because it is the first truly comprehensive, monumental work in this field. It does not deal just with cellular processes or just with clinical problems but with the entire spectrum of basic sciences and of lung function, metabolic functions, and respiratory defense mechanisms. The series will also include volumes that apply modern biological knowledge to elucidate mechanisms of pulmonary and respiratory disorders (immunologic, infectious, and genetic disorders, physiology and pharmacology of airways, genesis and resolution of pulmonary edema, and abnormalities of respiratory regulation). Other volumes will deal with the biology of specific pulmonary diseases (e.g., cancer, chronic obstructive pulmonary disease, disorders of the pulmonary circulation, and abnormalities associated with occupational and environmental factors) and with early detection and specific diagnosis.

This series shows the lung as a challenging organ, with many problems calling for innovative research. If it attracts some imaginative, creative, and perceptive young scientists to attack these difficult problems, the tremendous effort in writing, editing, and publishing these volumes will be well worthwhile. The volumes cannot win the Nobel Prize, but someone may who was challenged by them.

Julius H. Comroe, Jr.
San Francisco, California

PREFACE

Clinical interest in *Pneumocystis carinii* pneumonia in the United States is less than two decades old. I have decided that the most suitable preface would be a recollection of my personal introduction to this disease, and its effect on a professional career that has spanned this same interval.

In 1967, it was my privilege to join the Epidemic Intelligence Service of the National Centers for Disease Control in Atlanta, Georgia. I carpooled each morning to the CDC with Dr. Karl Western, a close friend with whom I had been a house officer. Karl's assignment was to work in the newly created Parasitic Diseases Drug Service, under the direction of Dr. Myron Schultz. The purpose of the service was to provide rarely used drugs in emergency situations to individuals who needed treatment for unusual parasitic disorders, most of which were contracted following overseas exposure. In the ensuing months, I learned from Karl of the newly recognized entity of *Pneumocystis carinii* pneumonia. This was a diffuse inflammatory process of the lungs apparently caused by an organism that no one could culture, but against which an anti-trypanasomal agent, pentamidine, had been used successfully to treat some human cases. On many occasions I recall seeing either Karl Western or Myron Schultz headed for the Atlanta post office to drop off emergency shipments of pentamidine to hospitals caring for individuals with hematologic malignancy or recipients of organ transplants. In those days, the disease came to be known as "transplant pneumonia" and it was often confused with cytomegalovirus infection of lung.

I followed the epidemiologic investigations of this disease with Karl Western during our two years at CDC, and appreciated, albeit secondhand, his experiences at St. Jude's Children Hospital in Memphis where pneumocystis was identified as one of the most common causes of pneumonia in leukemic children (Perera et al., 1970). He wagered me that in any series of diffused pneumonias of undetermined etiology, appropriate sectioning and staining of pulmonary tissue would reveal pneumocystis in a large proportion of cases. To diagnose pneumocystis infection, one first had to consider that it might be present and use the right technique to demonstrate the presence of cyst or trophozoite forms in lung tissue. Unless one knew what to search for, one would not establish the diagnosis.

Having been prepared at CDC, I soon became familiar with the protean clinical manifestations of *Pneumocystis carinii* infections in immunocompromised patients. In 1969, I moved to the Memorial Sloan-Kettering Cancer Center in New York for an infectious disease fellowship with Dr. Donald Armstrong. Many a patient with bizarre pulmonary processes that we did not understand turned out, sometimes too late for effective therapy, to have *Pneumocystis carinii* pneumonia. I remember vividly one patient who had normal chest x-rays but merely had severe dyspnea and hypoxia. Armstrong insisted on performing an open-lung biopsy in spite of absence of lung infiltrates. This in fact yielded the correct diagnosis of pneumocystis infection. The experience taught me to consider the diagnosis in the hypoxic immunosuppressed patient who lacks radiologic abnormalities on chest examination. This was ten years before this same type of presentation was noted in patients with pneumocystis complicating the acquired immunodeficiency syndrome (AIDS).

At Memorial, we encountered a dilemma which has confronted all clinicians who must deal with immunosuppressed patients that have diffuse lung infiltrates. Should we be aggressive and insist upon an invasive diagnostic procedure that has a high risk of complications? Or should we treat empirically with a potentially toxic drug like pentamidine and risk the consequences of empiric therapy? We could make an argument in those days that a negative lung biopsy would spare the patient the toxicity of pentamidine. Many clinicians, however, stubbornly resisted the idea of aggressive intervention, even though Walter Hughes, at the St. Jude's Children Cancer Research Hospital in Memphis, had repeatedly demonstrated the utility, efficacy, and safety of percutaneous transthoracic needle biopsies in children (Chaudhary et al., 1977). The latter technique proved less successful and certainly less safe in the adult population, but I personally became convinced that in the hands of a skilled surgeon, open-lung biopsy was a safe procedure and could be done even in intubated patients.

Moving to UCLA in the early 1970s presented me with an entirely different opportunity, namely, of following patients who were first being prepared, conditioned, and then treated in order to receive an allogeneic bone marrow transplant for the attempted cure of bone marrow aplasia or acute leukemia. The first results, particularly in leukemia, were extremely disappointing and we were confronted with myriad infectious complications. In retrospect it seems that we were transplanting patients far too late in the course of their disease when they already had established life-threatening infections which would progress explosively given the additional immunosuppression that is administered as part of the conditioning regimen. If the patient survived the acute post-transplant period we learned that pneumocystis was to become one of the most important post-transplant infectious complications. It was a common cause of interstitial pneumonia and could be confused with cytomegalovirus infection. Occasionally, as has been noted by many other clinicians, CMV and pneumocystis have occurred together. At about that time we heard of the important work of Walter Hughes and associates (1974), who extended the previous work of Dutz (1970) and Frenkel (Frenkel et al., 1966) in exploring the combined activity of folate antagonists with sulfonamides against murine pneumocystis. Encouraged by these reports we began to use trimethoprim/sulfamethoxazole in adult patients with documented disease. We were immediately confronted by a troublesome clinical dilemma so often encountered in the management of immunocompromised hosts. There was an existing, apparently effective therapy, namely pentamidine, that had been about 60% effective as reported by the CDC based on data returned to the Parasitic Diseases Drug Service (Walzer et al., 1976). Why jeopardize patient care and substitute an unproven medication like trimethoprim/sulfamethoxazole, which had only been successful in rats? Dare we risk human lives in an attempt to prove that the new treatment would be successful? There is no question that the most elegant work in the field of pneumocystis therapy and prophylaxis has been carried out by Hughes and his colleagues, who carefully managed a very well defined population at the St. Jude's Children's Cancer Research Hospital. These studies must rank among the most important ever carried out in the field of antimicrobial prophylaxis and treatment and are exemplary models of study design and analysis (Hughes, 1982). Our studies in the adult rather than the pediatric age population were less rigidly structured but gave the same encouraging results. We argued that the use of trimethoprim/sulfamethoxazole offered an alternative to a potentially toxic compound like pentamidine and that ease of administration by the oral route is a definite advantage (particularly for long-term prophylaxis). There were problems, nonetheless, with the oral preparation. Erratic absorption in some very ill patients led to low blood levels and clinical failure. Thus, we welcomed the subsequent development of parenteral trimethoprim/sulfamethoxazole. Meanwhile, as the evidence of the prophylactic efficacy of trimethoprim/sulfamethoxazole in leukemic children convinced all but the most skeptical. We also observed (in an uncontrolled study) the virtual eradication of pneumocystis infection in marrow transplants who were given intermittent post-transplant prophylaxis. By the year 1978, we found that *Pneumocystis carinii,* once a very important disease in our patient population, had virtually disappeared. We had concluded that therapy or prophylaxis was safe and well tolerated, therapeutic trials showed that it was as good if not better than pentamidine with fewer side effects, and that the combination was the treatment of choice for proven disease (Young, 1982).

So persuaded was I that pneumocystis had disappeared as an important clinical entity that we abandoned a number of research efforts initiated earlier in the decade. These included efforts to cultivate the parasite in vitro, the development of serodiagnostic techniques for measurement of human anticyst antibodies, and the study of interactions between cysts or trophozoites and phagocytic cells. Little did we suspect that just ahead of us would be the most important, and certainly the most well-publicized epidemic of pneumocystis infections ever documented in the history of medicine. It appears that this epidemic at the time of this writing shows no sign of abating. I refer, of course, to AIDS or Acquired Immunodeficiency Syndrome, wherein *Pneumocystis carinii* has been far and away the most common of the life-threatening opportunistic infections. A "crash program" of basic research has probably identified the causative viral agent (a retrovirus), but we do not have a chemotherapeutic means for treating this invariably fatal syndrome. The first few cases of pneumocystis in previously healthy homosexuals (first reported by Gottlieb from UCLA) (Gottlieb et al., 1981) were regarded as curiosities. After several hundred similar examples were reported in the United States, such cases no longer remained a joking matter. Suddenly *Pneumocystis carinii* was back in the medical headlines and governmental funding institutions expressed their willingness to support both basic research and a program to screen for more active compounds against this pathogen.

In the meantime, it has been noted by many observers that the available medications, particularly trimethoprim/sulfamethoxazole, did not seem to be working as well as in "conventional" immunosuppressed patients; a high incidence of allergic reactions was also noted. The most striking question about the current epidemic of pneumocystis in AIDS is "why is pneumocystis so common?" The evidence seems persuasive that pneumocystis is a universally acquired childhood infection, possibly one of the very many respiratory illnesses manifested by mild respiratory symptoms that most children have and can overcome in their younger years. The thesis currently accepted is that clinical disease represents reactivated infection occurring in patients with severely compromised cell-mediated immunity. Yet the question still remains, why pneumocystis as a cause of pneumonitis and why not a host of other organisms (viral, parasitic, or even bacterial) that remain latent in the host after an initial encounter. While I had intended this book to be a survey of the "state of the art" to supplement the last major review in 1976 (Robbins et al., 1976), I believe there are far more questions now about the pathogenesis of pneumocystis in AIDS that need to be addressed. Yet the patient material remains difficult to obtain, the diagnosis is challenging to establish, and many of the old problems that were faced 15 years ago at the start of the Parasitic Diseases Drug Service at the CDC persist.

The fascinating story of *Pneumocystis carinii* infections in man has no happy ending. It emphasizes that some medical problems certainly defy solution and may assume new guises. The irony is that we had effective therapy and prophylaxis for a few years in the 1970s without knowing how the microbe propagates. The early treatment data with several chemotherapeutic agents is a tribute to empiricism in medicine rather than to an approach to disease management based on careful understanding of parasite biology. I am not suggesting that empiricism should reign in our desperate search for new antipneumocystis compounds. I would emphasize in closing that persistence of pneumocystis infections in this day and age, indeed its growing challenge, emphasizes the need for long-range research planning and the need for basic investigations aimed at obtaining a better understanding of microbes and their interaction with host defenses. If AIDS were to mysteriously disappear within the next few years, we should not abandon the pursuit of new knowledge about pneumocystis or other troublesome pathogens that complicate AIDS. Knowledge of the mechanisms of intracellular parasites and the factors affecting conversion from the latent state to active infection should be a high priority in pneumocystis research just as it is with the study of herpesvirus infections which often appear concurrently.

Lowell S. Young

References

Chaudhary, S., Hughes, W. T., Feldman, S., Sanyal, S. K., Coburn, T., Ossi, M., and Cox, F. (1977). Percutaneous transthoracic needle aspiration of the lung. *Am. J. Dis. Child.* **131**:902.

Dutz, W. (1970). *Pneumocystis carinii* pneumonia. *Pathol. Annual* **5**:309.

Frenkel, J. K., Good, J. T., and Shultz, J. A. (1966). Latent pneumocystis infection of rats, relapse and chemotherapy. *Lab. Invest.* **15**:1559.

Gottlieb, M. S., Schroff, R., and Schanker, H. M. (1981). *Pneumocystis carinii* pneumonia and mucosal candidiasis in previously healthy homosexual men: Evidence of a new acquired cellular immunodeficiency. *N. Engl. J. Med.* **301**:1425.

Hughes, W. T. (1982). Trimethoprim-sulfamethoxazole therapy for *Pneumocystis carinii* pneumonitis in children. *Rev. Infect. Dis.* **4**:602.

Hughes, W. T., McNabb, P. C., Makres, T. D., et al. (1974). Efficacy of trimethoprim and sulfamethoxazole in the prevention and treatment of *Pneumocystis carinii* pneumonitis. *Antimicrobs. Agents Chemother.* **5**:289.

Perera, D. R., Western, K. A., Johnson, H. D., Johnson, W. W., Shultz, M. G., and Akers, P. V. (1970). *Pneumocystis carinii* pneumonia in a hospital for children. *JAMA* **214**:1074.

Robbins, J. B., DeVita, V. T., and Dutz, W. (Eds.). (1976). *Symposium on Pneumocystis carinii Infection NCI Monograph #43.* Washington, National Cancer Institute.

Walzer, P. D., Perl, D. P., Krogstad, D. J., Rawson, P. G., and Schultz, M. G. (1976). *Pneumocystis carinii* pneumonia in the United States: Epidemiology, diagnostic, and clinical features. In *Symposium on Pneumocystis carinii Infection. NCI Monograph #43.* Edited by J. B. Robbins, V. T. DeVita, Jr., and W. Dutz. Washington, National Cancer Institute, p. 55.

Young, L. S. (1982). Treatment of *Pneumocystis carinii* in adults with trimethoprim/sulfamethoxazole. *Rev. Infect. Dis.* **4**:608.

INTRODUCTION

Despite the discovery of penicillin in 1940, and of a myriad of other antibiotics since then, infections of the respiratory tract remain among the most important public health problems. They rank fifth as a cause of death and are virtually first as a cause of morbidity.

Pneumococcus was the first respiratory infectious agent to be identified. This was slightly more than 100 years ago. Many other agents have sebsequently been discovered, and each has posed scientists and physicians with a unique challenge to which they responded with enthusiasm and often with much success.

This volume addresses a pulmonary infection that has generated much interest for over 70 years. Indeed it was shortly after the beginning of this century that *Pneumocystis carinii* or its predecessor was described by Chagas and then by Carini. Our knowledge about this disease has evolved in successive phases. First, great strides were made to uncover its pathology, then it was recognized that immunodeficient patients or subjects receiving immunodepressive therapies were prime candidates for the disease. This led to the term "opportunistic infection."

It was, however, not until the discovery that *Pneumocystis carinii* is so often associated with Kaposi's sarcoma that this pathological entity received the attention that it warranted. Much has been written about it during the last few years, but no compendium is as comprehensive as this volume, edited by Dr. Lowell Young. Dr. Young brings to this book a lifelong experience in the study of *Pneumocystis carinii*. In addition, he has assembled a group of experts who add to the uniqueness of this monograph.

This volume is the 22nd in the series "Lung Biology in Health and Disease," but it is the first that focuses exclusively on a single disease, a disease of paramount importance today. We are, therefore, proud of the contribution this monograph makes to the series. Both personally and on behalf of all those who have contributed to the series, I express our gratitude to Dr. Young and his coauthors.

Claude Lenfant, M.D.
Bethesda, Maryland

xiii

CONTENTS

PNEUMOCYSTIS CARINII PNEUMONIA

1

Introduction and Historical Perspective

LOWELL S. YOUNG

University of California at Los Angeles
Center for the Health Sciences
Los Angeles, California

I. History and Background

The histologic diagnosis of pneumocystis infection is infrequently made in most hospitals, yet it is probably fair to state that this disease should be considered in the clinical evaluation of every immunodeficient patient who develops a pulmonary infiltrate. During the last 15 years, the presumed protozoan parasite *Pneumocystis carinii* has attracted clinical attention as the cause of a syndrome which is one of the most challenging diagnostic problems in the immunocompromised host. The early history of the disease, however, is most curious. The first identification of the morphologic forms that we now accept as pneumocysts is credited to Chagas, who published morphological studies of the lungs of guinea pigs experimentally infected with *Trypanosoma cruzi* (Dutz, 1970). A year later another Brazilian investigator, Carini, observed similar cysts in lungs of rats with experimental trypanosomiasis, but disputed Chagas' claim that the cystlike structures represented a sexual form of the American trypanosome (Ruskin, 1981). The species designation was credited to Carini by the Parisian workers, the Delanoes, who noted similar forms in the lungs of sewer rats. In 1913, Chagas also described in the autopsy of an adult, the first probably case of human pneumocystosis (Ruskin, 1981). However, no connection with human disease was made for many years thereafter. During and after the Second World War, conditions of malnutrition and overcrowding in orphanages in Europe were associated with epidemics of pneumonia. Histologically, the lungs of infants dying of epidemic pneumonia contained prominent plasma or round cell infiltration, and such cases became known as "interstitial plasma cell pneumonitis" of the epidemic type. Following World War II institutional outbreaks continued to occur in foundling homes in the Middle East where overcrowding and malnutrition were common. This phenomena still persists. Orphans brought to the United States from Southeast Asia have developed respiratory infections which have proven to be histologically documented examples of pneumocystis infection (Radman, 1973). Similarly, recent Haitian refugees subjected to conditions of malnutrition and overcrowding have developed pneumocystis pneumonia, along with other evidence of acquired immunodeficiency (Centers for Disease Control, 1982a).

II. *Pneumocystis carinii* in Immunosuppressed Hosts

Although the epidemics in foundling homes led to the epidemiologic and clinical investigations that established a firm basis for diagnosis and treatment of this disorder, the clinical syndrome that most modern clinicians are familiar with occurs in a relatively different group, immunosuppressed hosts. Gadjusek's work in 1957 established a firm association between pneumocystis infection and congenital immunodeficiency syndromes (Gadjusek, 1957). In addition to those patients with an inborn defect of antibody synthesizing capacity (B-cell disorder), those with impaired delayed hypersensitivity cellular (T-cell) mechanisms seem even more susceptible. A far larger group of subjects have acquired host defects secondary to development of a neoplasm such as Hodgkins disease or treatment with immunosuppressive therapy such as corticosteroids. In the 1980s, the most fascinating "new" presentation of pneumocystis infection has occurred in association with a homosexual lifestyle, drug abuse, and Kaposi's sarcoma (Gottlieb et al., 1981; Siegel et al., 1981). Epidemiologically, some of these cases have appeared in clusters, afflicted subjects have been apparently immunologically intact before onset of disease, but multiple immunologic abnormalities have been documented. Although a great deal of attention has focused on this syndrome, it has not been restricted to male homosexuals; multiply transfused patients with hemophilia A have had both pneumocystosis and evidence for acquired immunodeficiency, and there has been intense speculation about a provocative agent which could be transmitted by transfusions (Centers for Disease Control, 1982b). Thus, while the prime targets of pneumocystis infection in secondary and tertiary care hospitals are cancer patients and recipients of organ transplants who are usually given corticosteroid treatment, this infectious process has assumed yet other major forms of clinical presentation which have challenged those seeking to understand its pathogenesis, diagnosis, and treatment.

III. Cultivation

It has been equally frustrating that except for a few reports, long-term cultivation of this presumed parasite in high yield has not been accomplished. Koch's postulates have not been fulfilled for this disease, and the best evidence that *Pneumocystis* is an infectious entity is the presence of characteristic cyst forms in the lungs of humans and infected animals followed by their disappearance and clearing of pneumonitis after treatment with one of several chemotherapeutic agents. The appellation which the Delanoes gave to the cystlike forms that they observed in rat lung, *Pneumocystis carinii,* is technically appropriate only for the forms observed in rats (Frenkel, 1976). The strongest initial evidence linking the presence of cysts to human pneumonic disease was provided by Dr. Otto Jirovec and his associate, working in Prague during the 1940s (Vanek and Jirovec, 1952). In fact, Frenkel has argued that a more appropriate designation for the human strains should be *Pneumocystis jiroveci* (Frenkel, 1976). Since neither the rat nor the human strains have been cultivated in large number in vitro, definitive classification of these organisms by phenotypic and genotypic characteristics has not been possible. Nonetheless some evidence exists from the work of Walzer and Rutledge (1980) that, at least on the basis of antibody reactivity, the human and murine strains are different, and that has been our conclusion from unpublished studies as well. The dilemma faced by many who write about this disease is whether or not to continue to call the organism isolated from man *Pneumocystis carinii* or *Pneumocystis* species. For the sake of convention and familiarity, the clinical syndrome will still be referred to as *Pneumocystis carinii* pneumonia.

IV. Epidemiology and Diagnosis

Besides the problems with in vitro cultivation, there seem to be major gaps in our understanding about the epidemiology and noninvasive diagnosis of this disease. From the serologic studies of several centers, there is mounting evidence that pneumocystis infection is probably a common childhood infection that results in low levels of residual antibodies in the serum of many, if not most, normal adult subjects (Meuwissen et al., 1977). Attempts to use such immune responses, or the converse phenomena, the detection of antigen(s) circulating in the bloodstream of infected patients, have not met with consistent reproducible results. Antibody detection systems for diagnosis rely on measurement of a host humoral antibody response, but this is clearly impaired in many patients who are at risk of developing pneumocystis infection.

Paradoxically, in spite of the problems of understanding and diagnosing this infection short of an invasive and possibly dangerous surgical procedure, considerable progress has been made in the treatment and prophylaxis of this infection. From a situation in which *Pneumocystis* was one of the most common infections in childhood leukemia, an almost 100 percent reduction in the disease has followed prophylactic use of trimethoprim-sulfamethoxazole (Hughes et al., 1977). Clearly, this has been one of the most important achievements in the history of the disease. Nonetheless, the therapy of established infection is still challenging and the possibility of drug resistance cannot be evaluated with present laboratory techniques.

The Parasitic Diseases Drug Service of the Centers for Disease Control was the first to obtain important epidemiologic and therapeutic information for treatment of pneumocystis with pentamidine, the first widely studies agent that has proved effective against this pathogen (Western et al., 1970). While pentamidine has been largely supplanted by trimethoprim-sulfamethoxazole as initial therapy, it continues to be used in refractory cases and in patients with sulfonamide allergy. Indiscriminate use of antimicrobial agents which affect this pathogen or empiric use in cases of pneumonitis where the etiology is unknown may lead to drug resistance. Presently there are no reliable, readily available laboratory methods for monitoring drug resistance of this parasite.

Unquestionably, the single most valuable modern reference for pneumocystis infections is a monograph published in 1976 summarizing the proceedings of a symposium held at the National Cancer Institute in 1974 (Robbins et al., 1976). Since that time, important new information has been obtained about the epidemiology of pneumocystis infection and the important animal and in vitro work of Walzer (Walzer and Rutledge, 1980), Mazur, and their co-workers has appeared. New clinical syndromes involving pneumocystis infection have appeared and newer diagnostic and therapeutic approaches are available. Thus, it is the intention of this work to bring together much of the clinical and laboratory information about pneumocystis infection that has appeared since the National Cancer Institute Symposium. The hope that new chemotherapy and prophylaxis of this disease would lead to a reduction in the importance of this entity has been shortlived. *Pneumocystis carinii* remains an important, fascinating, pathogen in modern medical practice.

References

Center for Disease Control (1982b). Opportunistic Infections and Kaposi's sarcoma among Haitians in the United States. *Morbid. Mortal. Wkly. Rep.* **31**:353-354.

Center for Disease Control (1982b). *Pneumocystis carinii* pneumonia among persons with hemophilia A. *Morbid. Mortal. Wkly. Rep.* **31**:365-367.

Dutz, W. (1970). *Pneumocystis carinii* pneumonia. *Pathol. Ann.* **5**:309-341.

Frenkel, J. K. (1976). *Pneumocystis jiroveci* n. sp. In *Symposium on Pneumocystis carinii Infection NCI Monograph #43.* Edited by J. B. Robbins, V. T. DeVita Jr., and W. Dutz. Washington, National Cancer Institute, pp. 13-30.

Gajdusek, D. C. (1957). *Pneumocystis carinii*—etiologic agent of interstitial plasma cell pneumonia of young and premature infants. *Pediatrics* **19**: 543.

Gottlieb, M. S., Schroff, R., and Schanker, H. M. (1981). *Pneumocystis carinii* pneumonia and mucosal candidiasis in previously healthy homosexual men: Evidence of a new acquired cellular immunodeficiency. *N. Engl. J. Med.* **301**:1425-1430.

Hughes, W. T., Kuhn, S., Chaudhary, S., Feldman, S., Verzosa, M., Aur, R. J. A., Pratt, C., and Eorge, S. L. (1977). Successful chemoprophylaxis of *Pneumocystis carinii* pneumonitis. *N. Engl. J. Med.* **297**:1419-1426.

Meuwissen, J. H. E. T., Tauber, I., Leeuwenberg, A. D. E. M., Beckers, P. J. A., and Sieben, M. (1977). Parasitologic and serological observations of infection with pneumocystis in humans. *J. Infect. Dis.* **136**:43-49.

Radman, J. C. (1973). *Pneumocystis carinii* pneumonia in an adopted Vietnamese infant. *JAMA* **230**:1561-1563.

Robbins, J. B., DeVita, V. T., Jr., and Dutz, W. (Eds.). (1976). *Symposium on Pneumocystis carinii infection NCI Monograph #43.* Washington, National Cancer Institute.

Ruskin, J. (1981). Parasitic diseases in the compromised host. In *Clinical Approach to Infection in the Compromised Host.* Edited by R. H. Rubin and L. S. Young. New York, Plenum Press, pp. 269-334.

Siegal, F. P., Lopez, C., Hammer, G. S., Brown, A. E., Kornfeld, S. J., Gold, J., Hassett, J., Hirschmann, S. Z., Cunningham-Rundles, C., Adelsberg, B. R., Parham, D. M., Siegal, M., Cunningham-Rundles, S., and Armstrong, D. (1981). Severe acquired immunodeficiency in male homosexuals, manifested by chronic perianal ulcerative herpes simplex lesions. *N. Engl. J. Med.* **305**:1439-1444.

Vanek, J., and Jirovec, O. (1952). Parasitäre pneumonie. "Interstitielle" Plasma zell pneumonie der Frü geburten verursach durch *Pneumocystis carinii* 261. *Bakt. Orig.* **158**:120-127.

Walzer, P. D., and Rutledge, M. E. (1980). Comparison of rat, mouse, and human *Pneumocystis carinii* by immunofluorescence. *J. Infect. Dis.* **142**:449.

Western, K. A., Perera, D. R., and Schultz, M. G. (1970). Pentamidine isethionate in the treatment of *Pneumocystis carinii* pneumonia. *Ann. Int. Med.* **73**:695-702.

2

Experimental Models of *Pneumocystis carinii* Infections

PETER D. WALZER*

Lexington Veterans Administration Medical Center
and University of Kentucky College of Medicine
Lexington, Kentucky

I. Introduction

Pneumocystis carinii was first discovered by Chagas in his studies of American trypanosomiasis in Brazil (Chagas, 1909). He noted the organism in the lungs of guinea pigs experimentally infected with *Trypanosoma cruzi* and thought it was a variant of this protozoan. In 1910 Carini identified the organism in trapanosome-infected rats (Carini, 1910). Delanoe and Delanoe (1912, 1914) reviewed Carini's specimens and found identical organisms in the lung of rats in Paris not infected with trypanosomes. These authors proved conclusively that the organism was not a variant or special form of trypanosome, but represented an entirely new species. They proposed the name *Pneumocystis carinii* in honor of Dr. Carini.

Since that time *P. carinii* has been found to exist as a saprophyte in the lungs of a variety of animals in nature, including man (Walzer, 1977).

**Present affiliation:* Cincinnati Veterans Administration Medical Center and University of Cincinnati College of Medicine, Cincinnati, Ohio.

In all studies to date, pneumocystis organisms found in these animal species have been morphologically indistinguishable. However, it is unclear whether species or strain differences exist in the organism. The taxonomic position of *P. carinii* is also unsettled. The organism has been classified as a fungus by some investigators owing to its ultrastructural properties and affinity for certain fungal strains (e.g., methenamine silver) (Csillag, 1957; Minielly et al., 1969; Vavra and Kucera, 1970). Most workers have classified *P. carinii* as a protozoan because of other structural properties, resemblance to *Toxoplasma,* and sensitivity to antiparasitic agents (Frenkel et al., 1966; Gajdusek, 1957; Ham et al., 1971).

The life cycle of *P. carinii* has not been completely worked out. Most studies have involved morphologic examination of infected human or animal lungs (Barton and Campbell, 1967, 1969; Campbell, 1972; Frenkel, 1976; Gold et al., 1977; Price and Hughes, 1974; Shively et al., 1974; Sueishi et al., 1977; Vossen et al., 1978; Wang et al., 1970). The terminology used in defining the different forms of *P. carinii* presumes that the organism is a protozoan. On light microscopy the most numerous form is the "trophozoite," which is small (1-4 microns), pleomorphic and best identified by the Giemsa stain. Trophozoites often occur in clumps which makes quantitation difficult. The 5-7-micron "cyst" has a thick cell wall which is stained by methenamine silver. The cyst is the form most readily identified in histopathologic sections, and a variety of selective cell wall stains have been used for this purpose. On Giemsa stain, the cyst contains up to 8 smaller intracystic bodies of daughter forms termed "sporozoites." It is thought that the daughter forms emerge from the cyst and develop into trophozoites, some of which ultimately mature and form cysts and repeat the cycle. However, this theory is largely speculative and little is known about the basis of reproduction of division of the organism.

On electron microscopy the pleomorphic nature of the trophozoite is readily apparent; the organism has a nucleus, a few cytoplasmic organelles, and tubular extensions of the cytoplasm termed "filopodia." The cyst has a very thick cell wall or "pellicle" and intracystic bodies. Other forms of *P. carinii* have also been identified. An intermediate stage with a rather thin cell but no filopodia has been termed the "precyst." A fourth form of the organism termed "empty" or "crescent-shaped cyst" is thought to represent the cyst which remains after extrusion of the intracystic bodies.

The natural habitat of the *P. carinii* is the alveolus. The organism maintains an intimate relationship with a specific alveolar lining cell, the type 1 pneumocyte. The lack of detailed intracytoplasmic organelles and other features has led to the suggestion that *P. carinii* obtains nourishment from the type 1 pneumocyte and/or alveolar fluid by metabolizing low molecular weight substances (Barton and Campbell, 1969).

For many years *P. carinii* was little more than a medical curiosity. The organism was first associated with human disease when it was found to be the etiological agent of interstitial plasma cell pneumonia. This illness was first described by Ammich (1938) and ravaged Eastern and Central Europe following World War II (Gajdusek, 1957). It primarily afflicted infants in orphanages and foundling homes where overcrowding, prematurity, debilitation, and malnutrition abounded; if untreated, it had a mortality of 50%. Interstitial plasma cell pneumonia often occurred in explosive hospital outbreaks, and thus has been termed the "epidemic" for of *P. carinii* infection. On histopathologic examination, the lungs stained with hematoxylin and eosin exhibited a foamy vacuolated alveolar exudate and a dense plasma cell interstitial infiltrate. Van de Meer and Brug (1942) identified *P. carinii* in the lung sections of patients, but an etiologic relationship of the organism was not established until the work of Vanek and Jirovek (1952). Interstitial plasma cell pneumonia has largely declined in Europe with improved socioeconomic conditions, but has been found in other parts of the world (Dutz, 1970). Its occurrence in Vietnamese and other orphans in the United States (Hyun et al., 1966; Gleason et al., 1975) emphasizes the need for American physicians to be familiar with the clinical manifestations and to institute prompt diagnosis and treatment.

Over the past 20 years *P. carinii* has become recognized as an important cause of pneumonia in the immunocompromised host (Burke and Good, 1973; Walzer et al., 1973, 1974). Three types of patients have been afflicted: (1) Patients of all ages receiving immunosuppressive agents for the treatment of cancer (particularly lymphoreticular malignancies), organ transplantation, and a variety of other disorders. Corticosteroids have been the most common type of immunosuppressive agent used. (2) Children and infants with primary immunodeficiency disorders, particularly severe combined immunodeficiency, which has defects in B- and T-lymphocyte function, and (3) the recently described acquired immune deficiency syndrome (AIDS) (see Chap. 8).

The specific host-immune defects which predispose to infection by *P. carinii* are poorly understood, but, overall, impaired cellular immunity appears to be more important than impaired humoral immunity. It is thought that in patients receiving immunosuppressive agents the mechanism of disease is reactivation of latent infection; the subclinical carrier state of *P. carinii* increases as more intensive immunosuppression is used (Perera et al., 1970). Malnutrition appears to be an important predisposing host factor (Hughes et al., 1974a) but other defects (e.g., in local antibody or complement system) remain poorly defined. The development of pneumocystis pneumonia after tapering of corticosteroid dose or immunological reconstitution by bone marrow transplantation (Rifkind et al., 1966; Solberg et al., 1971) raises the possibility of host inflammatory response in the production of clinical disease. The occurrence of institutional or hospital outbreaks or pneumocystis pneumonia even in populations of immunosuppressed patients (Ruebush et al., 1978; Singer et al., 1975) suggests the possibility of contagion.

II. Development of Animal Models

The occurrence of *P. carinii* in animals bears many similarities to the human condition. The organism usually exists as an incidental finding in lungs without eliciting host inflammatory response (Kucera, 1967; Lainson and Shaw, 1975; Poelma, 1975; Poelma and Broekhuizen, 1972; Sheldon, 1959a). Cases of frank pneumocystis pneumonia have been reported in goats, dogs, horses, swine, and primates without the use of immunosuppressive agents (Chandler et al., 1967; Copland, 1974; Farrow et al., 1972; Long et al., 1975; McClure et al., 1974; McConnell et al., 1971; Nicolskii and Shchetinin, 1967; Shively et al., 1973; Vanden Akker and Goldblood, 1960). Pathologic features and familial clustering of these cases suggest that an underlying immunodeficiency disease may have been present.

Studies of pneumocystis infection with animal models have been geared toward the use of immunosuppressive agents, primarily corticosteroids. The principal experimental animal has been the rat. Weller in 1955 found that pneumocystis pneumonia could be produced in rats inoculated with human-derived organisms and treated with corticosteroids and penicillin (Weller, 1956a, 1956b). Since pneumocystis pneumonia also occurred in uninoculated control rats treated with steroids and penicillin, he concluded that the pneumonia occurred by reactivation of latent infection. Similar results were found by several other workers (Goetz and Rentsch, 1957; Higuchi et al., 1972; Linhartova, 1956, 1958; Nakai and Kamata, 1974; Pliess and Trode, 1958; Ricken and Remington, 1967; Yoshida et al., 1974). In studies of the effects of corticosteroids in different animal species, Frenkel et al. (1963) found a high frequency of *P. carinii* pneumonia in rats. These investigators then set out to systematically study the rat model to determine the optimal steroid dose and preparation, to evaluate other immunosuppressive agents, to attempt experimental transmission of the organism, to devise new modes of treatment, and to prevent superinfection with other agents in these immunosuppressed animals (Frenkel et al., 1966). In the basic regimen, rats weighing 200 g were administered 25 mg subcutaneous cortisone acetate twice weekly, ate a regular diet, and drank tap water containing chlortetracycline. The chlortetracycline was used because steroid-treated rats have a high frequency of infection with *Corynebacterium kutscheri.*

The model developed by Frenkel has been widely used with minor modifications in studies of experimental *P. carinii* infection. Male outbred Sprague-Dawley rats have usually been used, but other strains work quite satisfactorily. The steroid dose or preparation can be varied depending upon experimental purposes; Hendley and Weller (1971), for example, used dexamethasone in the drinking water. Other tetracycline preparations can be substituted for the chlortetracycline without noticeable effect. In some instances, amphotericin B has been used to suppress fungal infection (Chandler et al., 1979), but in most cases fungal infection has not been a major problem.

The cortisone regimen is usually administered for about 8-12 weeks. The lungs slowly fill with *Pneumocystis* organisms. The hematoxylin and eosin-stained alveoli display the typical foamy eosinophilic material, whereas the interstitial inflammatory response is mild and nonspecific. This histopathological picture closely resembles the sporadic form of the pneumocystis pneumonia in the immunocompromised host rather than the epidemic form in the institutionalized infants. Methenamine silver-stained lung sections show typical masses of organisms. This model has been used extensively in light and electron microscopic studies and to develop new therapeutic modalities (Hughes et al., 1973, 1974b; Kluge et al., 1978; Western et al., 1975).

An important but not well publicized limitation of the steroid-treated rat model is the variation in the intensity of *P. carinii* pneumonia achieved. One group of rats obtained from a dealer may display heavy infection, whereas another group of the same type of rat obtained from the same dealer at a different time and administered the same steroid dose may display only light infection. This variation in intensity of infection may have some adverse effects on experimental studies. Hughes has found that a low (8%) protein diet enhances the intensity of steroid-induced *P. carinii* infection (Hughes et al., 1974a), however, this diet is quite expensive and has not been widely used.

III. Recent Studies in the Corticosteroid Treated Rat

In collaboration with Drs. Kokichi Yoneda and Ralph Powell, at the Lexington Veterans Administration Medical Center and University of Kentucky, the author initiated a series of studies to reexamine the rat *P. carinii* model (Gottschall et al., 1979; Walzer et al., 1979, 1980; Yoneda and Walzer, 1980, 1981; Yoneda et al., 1982). In preliminary experiments we were impressed with the regularity and intensity of *P. carinii* infection achieved when a low-protein diet was added to the corticosteroid regimen; thus, we employed this combination in our studies. The goals of these studies were:

1. To develop methods of quantitating *P. carinii* organisms in the lungs.

2. To correlate the changes in numbers of organisms with histopathologic events in the host lungs over time.

3. To study the long-term effect in the lungs after corticosteroids had been tapered.

Adult Sprague-Dawley rats weighing about 250 g were divided into three groups (Walzer et al., 1980). Group A rats (controls) received no steroids, ate a regular diet, and drank tap water with or without tetracycline (1 mg/ml). Group B rats received the standard treatment regimen of cortisone acetate (25 mg) injected subcutaneously twice weekly, a low-(8%) protein diet, and tetracycline in their drinking water for 8-9 weeks or until death. Group C rats received the standard regimen for 4 weeks; then a regular diet was substituted and the steroid dose was tapered to zero over the next 3 weeks. Thus, by week 7, all steroids had been discontinued. The rats were weighed at weekly intervals; varying numbers of rats from each group were sacrificed each week, their lungs were processed for histopathology, and serum was obtained by cardiac puncture. As seen in Figure 1, group A rats appeared healthy and increased their mean weight by 40-45% in 8 weeks. Group B rats became chronically ill and debilitated and lost 35% of their original weight. Few of these rats survived beyond 8 weeks. Group C rats lost weight during the first 4 weeks; their weights plateaued with steroid tapering and they slowly regained their original weight.

A standardized procedure was devised for grading the intensity of *P carinii* infection in lung sections, and was evaluated in both rats and mice. At least 3 blocks of lung tissue were removed for histopathologic examination: one from the upper and lower portions of the right lung and one from the midportion of the left lung. The lung sections were stained with methenamine silver, coded, and read blindly. The following scoring system for infection was used: 0, no *P. carinii* found; 0.5+, minimal infection $< 1\%$ alveoli involved; 1+, light, 1-25% alveoli involved; 2+, moderate, 25-50% alveoli involved; 3+, heavy, 50-75% alveoli involved; 4+, very heavy, $> 75\%$ alveoli involved.

For quantitation, portions of both lungs of a rat or a mouse were pooled and cut into small pieces, air dried, weighed, ground through a no. 60 wire mesh screen, digested with 0.2% collagenase and 0.2% hyaluronidase, washed, and resuspended in 1 ml of Hanks' balanced salt solution. Two 1 μl-drops of this material were placed on a slide, air dried, and stained with cresyl echt violet (CEV). This selectively stains the cell wall of *P. carinii* cysts (Bowling ct al., 1973). All cysts within each drop were counted and the mean count was taken as the cyst count per microliter; the number of cysts per milliliter, and, based on weight of the lung, the number of cysts per gram of lung tissue was then calculated. Quantitation of *P. carinii* was

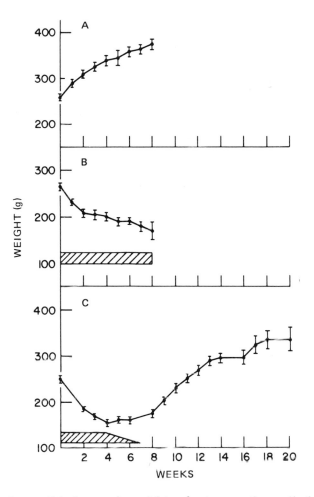

Figure 1 Sequential changes in weights of rats over time. Each point repre sents the mean + 1 SEM weight of the group of rats. Group A, controls. Group B, standard treatment regimen of corticosteroids (represented by hatch marks) low protein diet, and tetracycline in the drinking water. Group C, standard treatment regimen for 4 weeks, then placed on regular diet and tapering doses of steroids (hatch marks). (From Walzer et al., 1980.)

done both in rat and mouse lungs, and the results were then compared with the semiquantitative *P. carinii* score (Fig. 2). Using nonparametric statistics, a highly significant ($P < 0.001$) correlation was found between quantitative cyst count and histologic score for both rat and mouse lungs.

Quantitation by Giemsa stain, which identified both *P. carinii* cysts and trophozoites, was unsatisfactory. The trophozoites were small, occurred in clumps, and were often confused with tissue debris or platelets. Mature cyst forms were easily recognizable, but intermediate forms were often difficult to distinguish from other host cells. When compared with CEV stain, Giemsa stain yielded an underestimate of number of cysts.

The growth characteristics of *P. carinii* in the lungs are shown in Figure 3. Some group A control rats had minimal infection at the start of the study, consistent with the subclinical-clinical carrier state in nature. The tendency to acquire the infection did not appear to increase over time, and was not affected by the presence of tetracycline in the drinking water. The intensity of *P. carinii* infection in group B rats slowly progressed over time; it was light to moderate by 4 weeks and was very heavy by 7-8 weeks. The intensity of *P carinii* invection in group C rats did not diminish in the early weeks after discontinuation of steroids. These rats remained moderately infected through 13 weeks (i.e., 6 weeks after all steroids had been stopped), after which infection was classified as minimal because organisms stained by methenamine silver were few in number and had lost their characteristic morphology. However, even at 21 weeks, rare clusters of well-preserved organisms were seen.

The sequential changes of *P. carinii* in the lungs by light microscopy are shown in Figures 4a and 4b. In minimal or light infections, organisms were found in small numbers along alveolar walls. As the infection developed, more alveoli became involved and filled with clumps of organisms. In rats dying from *P. carinii,* alveoli were virtually filled with masses of pneumocystis organisms. In hematoxylin- and eosin-stained lung sections, there was the classic foamy eosinophilic material within alveoli. The host response was characterized by hypertrophy of alveolar lining cells (Fig. 5), slight prominence of alveolar macrophages, and a mild mononuclear cell interstitial infiltrate. With tapering of corticosteroids, alveolar macrophages became much more prominent and some multinucleated forms were observed. Hypertrophy of alveolar lining cells continued. The most striking changes found with steroid tapering were in the pulmonary interstitium. There was a lymphocytic infiltrate which was quite prominent by 9-10 weeks and reached peak intensity at 15-21 weeks (Fig. 6). The other change was the development of interstitial fibrosis, which was seen on both hematoxylin and eosin and on trichrome stains. The fibrosis first appeared at 9-10 weeks and progressively increased over time.

On electron microscopy *P. carini* trophozoites appeared much more

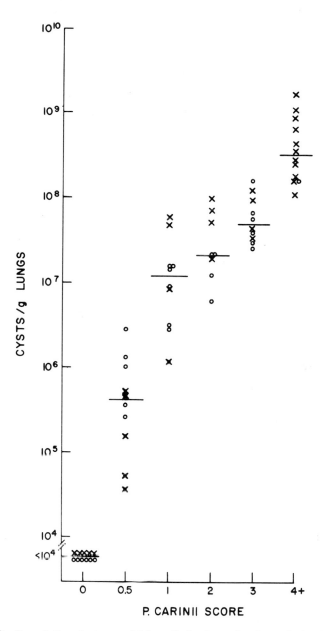

Figure 2 Correlation between histopathologic evaluation of the intensity of *P. carinii* infection and quantitative cyst count for rats (X) and (○). The horizontal bars represent median cyst counts. (From Walzer et al., 1980.)

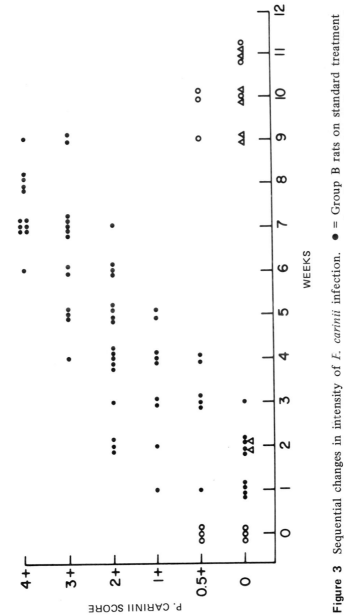

Figure 3 Sequential changes in intensity of *P. carinii* infection. ● = Group B rats on standard treatment regimen. ○ = Group A rats (control) which drank plain tap water. △ = Group A (control) rats that drank water with tetracycline. (From Walzer et al., 1980.)

numerous than the cysts; both forms of the organism progressively increased in number over time and gradually filled alveoli. Throughout the period of steroid administration in group B rats, the trophozoites lined alveolar walls, in close apposition to type 1 pneumocytes. The relationship of the tropozoites to type 1 pneumocytes was studied by the glycocalyx stain, Ruthenium red. Heavy deposits of stain were found on the alveolar surfaces of, but not between, the trophozoites and type 1 cells, indicating a rather tight apposition of the cell membranes (Fig. 7). Despite the close interaction of *P. carinii* and type 1 cells, morphologic changes in type 1 cells were not evident until the 7th week of steroid administration. At this time the degenerative changes appeared, characterized first by subepithelial bleb formation. The alveolar surface then became partially denuded in a fenestrated fashion. By 8 weeks the trophozoites covered the denuded alveolar epithelial surface and were in direct contact with the basement membrane. A few trophozoites were seen in the pulmonary interstitium.

Type 2 pneumocytes displayed a progressive increase in cellular volume and in the size of lamellar bodies over time. These hypertrophic changes were also observed in uninfected control rats drinking tap water containing a tetracycline. Such type 2 cell changes, which were even more pronounced in rats ingesting oxytetracycline than in rats ingesting generic tetracycline, are the subject of a separate study (Gottschall et al., 1979). Alveolar macrophages increased slightly in number over time in group B rats, but did not display any noticeable morpholocial changes.

The electron microscopic changes paralleled the light microscopic findings in group C rats with corticosteroid tapering. Trophozoites could still be found attached to type 1 cells at 21 weeks. No degenerative changes in type 1 pneumocytes were seen, but there was hypertrophy of type 2 cells. Alveolar macrophages increased in number and became more prominent in the phagocytosis of *P. carinii* (Fig. 8).

These studies demonstrate that *P. carinii* grows slowly in vivo in a manner which can be quantitated. Counting the number of cysts underestimates the total number of organisms, but cyst quantitation by the use of selective cell wall stains (methenamine silver, toluidine blue, CEV) is the most reliable marker for the number of *Pneumocystis* organisms in lung preparations. The major pitfall in cyst quantitation is the variation in the intensity of staining. In these studies, cyst counts increased from $\leqslant 10^4$ cysts (the minimal level of detection) to 10^9 cysts per gram of lung tissue at the peak level of infection at 7-8 weeks. Using somewhat different techniques Ogino (1978) and Ikai et al., (1977) have also demonstrated an increase in *P. carinii* cyst counts over time in steroid-treated rats. Thus, it may be possible to develop crude in vivo growth curves for *P. carinii*.

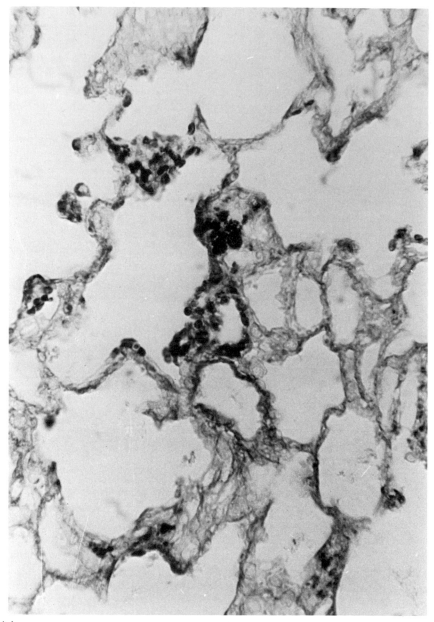

(a)

Figure 4 Sequential histologic changes in *P. carinii* infection.   Methenamine silver stain.   (a) Light-moderate *P. carinii* infection at 4 weeks of steroids (×500).

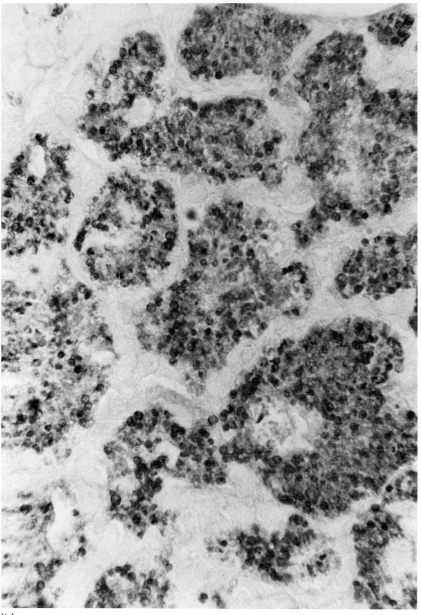

(b)

Figure 4 (continued) (b) Very heavy *P. carinii* infection in rat that died at 8 weeks of steroids. Note alveoli are virtually filled by masses of organisms (×500). (From Walzer et al., 1980.)

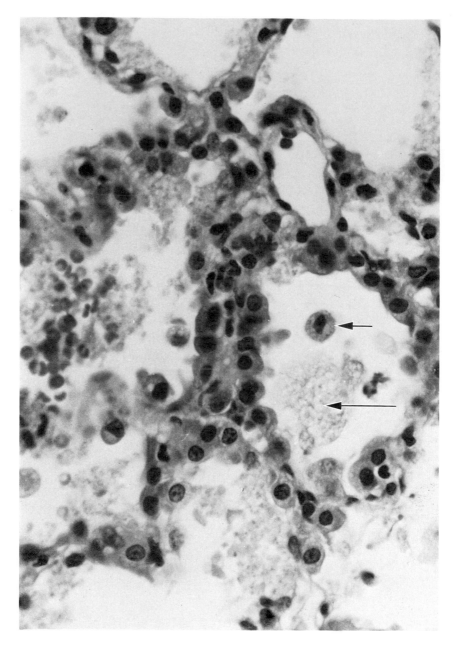

Figure 5 Hypertrophic alveolar lining cells are prominent along alveolar walls of rat sacrificed after 9 weeks of full doses of corticosteroids. Within alveolar lumens are foamy exudate (long arrow) and alveolar macrophages (short arrow). (Hematoxylin and eosin, ×620.) (From Walzer et al., 1980.)

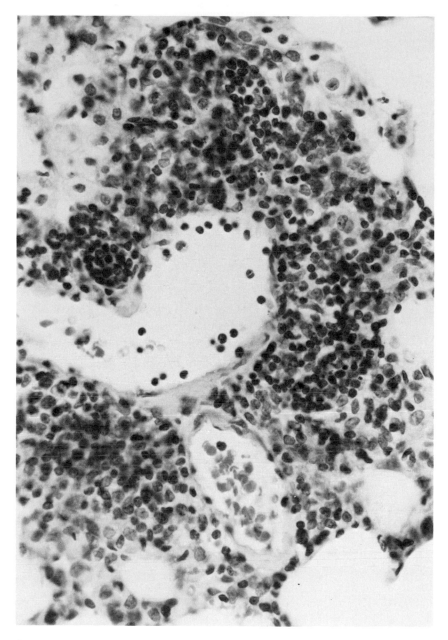

Figure 6 Mononuclear cell infiltrate in interstitial space surrounding small vessels of rat sacrificed after 15 weeks. (Hematoxylin and eosin, ×400.) (From Walzer et al., 1980.)

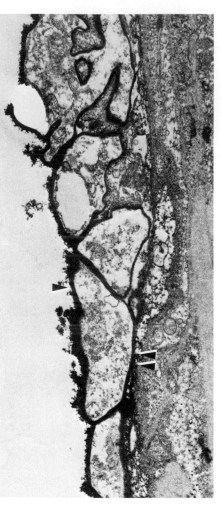

Figure 7 Alveolar surface at 7 weeks. Heavy stain deposits of Ruthenium red are seen on the alveolar surface of trophozoite and type I pneumocyte (arrow). Notice the absence of stain between the trophozoites and type I pneumocytes where they are attached (double arrow). Also notice the extension of type I pneumocyte cytoplasm between the trophozoites. (Ruthenium red stain ×15,000.) (From Yoneda and Walzer, 1980.)

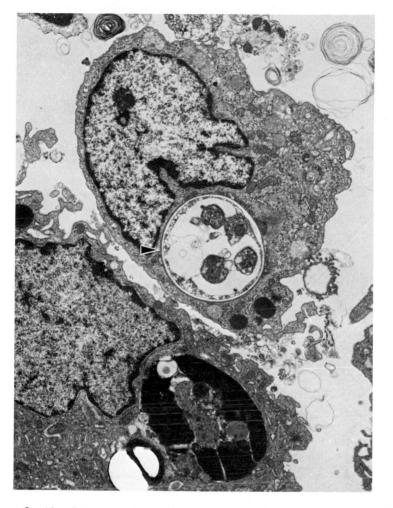

Figure 8 Alveolar macrophage after corticosteroids had been tapered (12th week of study). Notice intracellular *P. carinii* cyst, ×8500. (From Yoneda and Walzer, 1980.)

The interaction of *P. carinii* with the type 1 cell occupies a central role in the host-parasite relationship in this infection, and the first step in this process is that of organism attachment. Some authors have suggested that *P. carinii* attaches to the type 1 cell by filopodia (Barton and Campbell, 1969). We have not been able to confirm this, and our more recent data using freeze-fracture electron microscopy suggest that *P. carinii* attaches in an unusual manner (Yoneda and Walzer, 1983). The fact that degenerative changes in type 1 cells coincided with the peak intensity of *P. carinii* infection and the lack of such changes in a variety of control animals outlined in the study (Yoneda and Walzer, 1980) support the hypothesis that *P. carinii* can damage host cells. Similar findings have been reported recently by Lanken et al. (1980) in the rat model. The mechanism of this alveolar injury is unknown. The foamy eosinophilic material seen on light microscopy represents serum proteins, degenerative membranes of organism and host, and myelin figures considered to be pulmonary surfactant. The denuded basement membrane appears to be the site of exudation of fibrin and other serum proteins into the alveolus, and thus seems important in the formation of the eosinophilic material.

The presence of *P. carinii* in pulmonary interstitium raises the possibility of tissue invasion of the organism, probably through the denuded basement membrane. Spread of *P. carinii* beyond the lungs has rarely been reported in humans, such findings are primarily in patients with primary immunodeficiency disorders (Walzer, 1977). In limited autopsy surveys, the presence of *P. carinii* outside the lungs has also been infrequent (Price and Hughes, 1974; Barnett et al., 1969). On the other hand, the possibility of intrauterine transmission of *P. carinii* and the role of the organism as a cause of pneumonia in newborns has been raised (Bazaz et al., 1970; Pavlica, 1962; Stagno et al., 1980). Ogino did not find *P. carinii* outside the lungs in steroid-treated rats (Ogino, 1978), and limited studies of our own rats support these conclusions. However, since so little is known about the biology and life cycle of *P. carinii,* the possibility of spread beyond the lungs remains an intriguing question. This can probably best be answered by developing animal models which can be infected with exogenous *P. carinii,* and by using more sensitive techniques than simple light microscopy, which has been used in studies up to now, to look for extrapulmonary organisms.

The hypertrophy of type 2 cells seen on both light and electron microscopy is a typical host response to alveolar damage. It would be nice to conclude that this hypertrophy was secondary to changes in the type 1 cells, but the presence of hypertrophy in uninfected control rats that injested tetracycline made such an interpretation premature. The substitution of other antibiotics in the drinking water might help clarify this question.

The slow clearance of *P. carinii* from the lungs with corticosteroid tapering was due, at least in part, to the rather profound effects of the combination of steroids and protein calorie malnutrition. In the only comparable study Frenkel et al. (1966) administered regular diet and steroids to rats for 5 weeks and then abruptly withdrew the steroids; after 3 weeks, *P. carinii* had been almost completely cleared from the lungs. In our study the presence of *P. carinii* at 21 weeks suggested that the organism is present as a latent infection long after normal immune function has been restored. Recently Hughes found that prolonged treatment with trimethoprim-sulfamethoxazole failed to eradicate *P. carinii* completely from the lungs (Hughes, 1979). These data and the fact that in vitro studies suggest that trimethoprim-sulfamethoxazole may not be cidal to *P. carinii* (Pesanti, 1980) have important clinical implications. Any chemoprophylaxis program must take into account that *P. carinii* may remain a latent infection once the drug is stopped, even if normal immune function has been restored.

The role of alveolar macrophages in host defense mechanism against *P. carinii* is unclear, and is discussed in greater detail elsewhere in this book. Macrophages did not prevent the proliferation of *P. carinii* during corticosteroid administration; however, when steroids were discontinued, alveolar macrophages became quite active in the phagocytosis of *P. carinii*. Some in vitro studies have shown that opsonizing antibody is necessary for phagocytosis of *P. carinii* by alveolar macrophages (Masur and Jones, 1978), whereas other studies performed under different cultural conditions have shown that phagocytosis may occur in the absence of the antibody (Von Behren and Pesanti, 1978). More studies are needed in the area of macrophage-lymphocyte interaction to learn about host-defense mechanisms in this infection.

The most dramatic changes in host inflammatory responses to corticosteroid tapering were the development of interstitial lymphocytic infiltrate and fibrosis. The relationship of interstitial fibrosis to *P. carinii* infection has been a matter of controversy. Fibrosis has been observed in some patients and in a few rats with pneumocystis pneumonia (Frenkel et al., 1966; Price and Hughes, 1974; Rosen et al., 1972; Von Behren and Pooanti, 1978; Weber et al., 1977; Whitcomb et al., 1970). Since patients often receive a variety of other substances which can damage the lung (e.g., oxygen, cancer chemotherapy, radiation), or may have infection with another organism, the role of *P. carinii* in these changes is not clear. In our rat model, the increase in fibrosis over time and its correlation with other host inflammatory changes and clearance of *P. carinii* from the lung support the hypothesis that recovery from this infection may be associated with interstitial fibrosis.

These studies do not address the question of why patients seem to develop pneumocystis pneumonia when steroids are being tapered. It may be, that in this instance, the rat model does not mimic the human condition. Rats have been classified "steroid-sensitive" species whereas humans are "steroid-resistant" (Claman, 1972). On the other hand, it may be that the human condition is analogous to the situation in the rat, since the intensity of *P. carinii* infection increased initially after steroid tapering. The organism multiplied slowly, and steroid effects remained in the rats for a long time after injections had been stopped.

These studies may have relevance to other pulmonary conditions. Degeneration of type 1 cells is considered to be a nonspecific reaction to injury from a variety of agents. *Pneumocystis carinii* infection may provide a new model to study the degeneration process because of the slow evolution of the changes. Hypertrophy of type 2 cells is a host reparative phenomenon to injury from a variety of agents. Hypertrophy secondary to tetracyclines is independent of any alveolar injury, and thus could serve as a model system to study type 2 cell function.

We have also conducted electron microscopic studies of the interaction of *P. carinii* with host type 1 cells during the period before the appearance

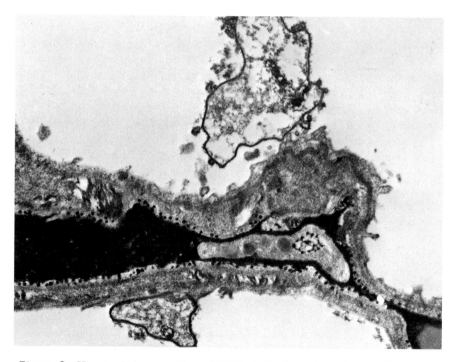

Figure 9 Horseradish peroxidase (HRP) study in a 4 week experiment rat. HRP is confined in the vascular space. ×8500. (From Yoneda and Walzer, 1981.)

of degenerative changes in the type 1 cell (Yoneda and Walzer, 1981). It was thought that these changes might be secondary to pulmonary edema, and thus, possibly due to alterations in the permeability of the alveolar capillary membrane. Using horseradish peroxidase as an ultrastructural marker, group B steroid-treated rats were studies at 4 weeks when *P. carinii* was firmly attached to type 1 cells. Uninfected rats not receiving steroids served as controls. As can be seen in Figure 9, horseradish peroxidase injected intravenously into rats was confined to the intravascular space in rats treated for 4 weeks with steroids and in control rats. By contrast, in rats treated for 7 weeks with steroids, horseradish peroxidase leaked out of vascular space into the interstitium, and eventually into the alveolar space (Fig. 10). This fluid accumulation between the type 1 cells was responsible for the subepithelial bleb formation, the first manifestation of changes in host cells to *P. carinii* infection. Thus, the primary injury in *P. carinii* infection appears to be in-

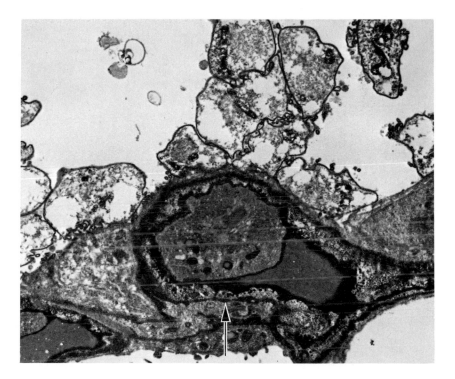

Figure 10 HRP study in a 7-week experiment rat. HRP is seen in the vascular space, intercellular space of the endothelium and in the basement membrane (arrow). (×8500.) (From Yoneda and Walzer, 1981.)

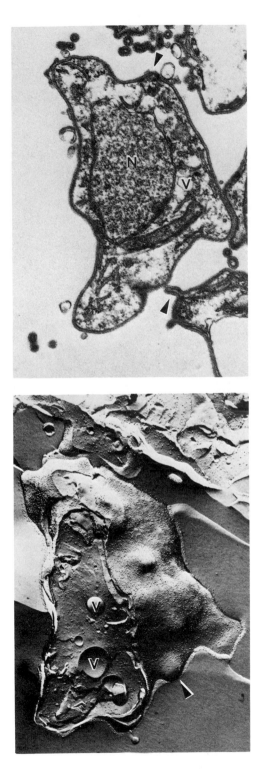

Figure 11a Thin-section photograph of a trophic organism. Notice the irregular shape, a central nucleus (N) and mitochondria, and a few vacuoles (V), filopodia (arrow) are seen stretching from the cell body. (Uranyl acetate and lead citrate stain, ×28,000.) (From Yoneda et al., 1982.)

Figure 11b Freeze-fracture image of a trophic organism. Notice two layers of the pellicle. Filopodia (arrow) can be seen as bulges of cytoplasm. The smoothness of the vacuolar wall (V) is evident. (×28,000.) (From Yoneda et al., 1982.)

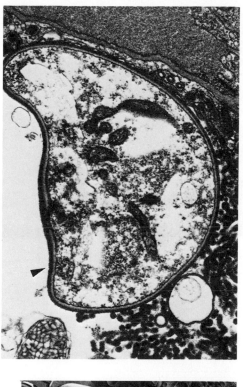

Figure 12a Thin section photograph of a precyst organism. Notice tightly packed outer layer of the cell wall. ($\times$ 19,000.) (From Yoneda et al., 1982.)

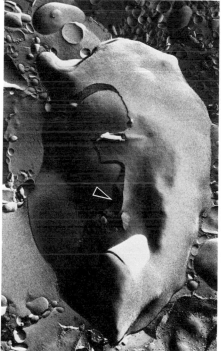

Figure 12b Freeze-fracture image of a precyst organism. Notice the smoothness of the surface and thickness of the wall (arrow). ($\times$ 19,000.) (From Yoneda et al., 1982.)

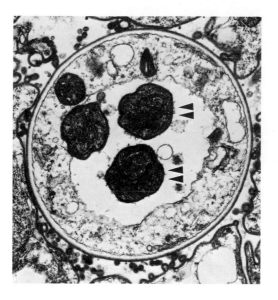

Figure 13a Thin-section photograph of a cyst. Notice the tightly packed wall and intracystic bodies (double arrow). (Uranyl acetate and lead citrate stain, ×16,000.) (From Yoneda et al., 1982.)

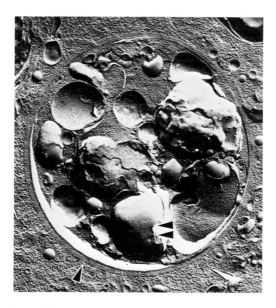

Figure 13b Freeze-fracture image of a cyst. The fracture plane crossed the center of the cyst. Notice the tightly packed wall (arrow) and intracystic bodies (double arrow). (×16,000.) (From Yoneda et al., 1982.)

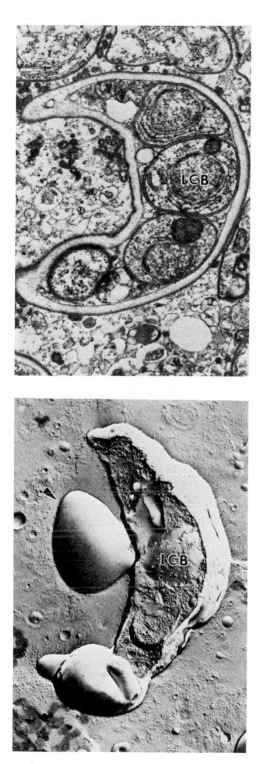

Figure 14a Thin-section photograph of a crescent-shaped cyst. Notice intracystic bodies (ICB). (Uranyl acetate and lead citrate stain, ×18,000.) (From Yoneda er al., 1982.)

Figure 14b Freeze-fractured crescent-shaped cyst. Two IBCs are seen within. Notice the smooth surface of the attached parts (arrow). (×18,000.) (From Yoneda et al., 1982.)

creased permeability of the alveolar-capillary membrane. The mechanism of this change is unclear, but a number of hypotheses can be offered: (a) a direct effect of *P. carinii* on the type 1 cell, as has been observed with cytomegalovirus infection (Brody et al., 1978); (2) soluble factors from *P. carinii;* or (3) perhaps changes in the pulmonary surfactant layer secondary to attachment to *P. carinii* to the type 1 cell.

Our other studies have employed ultrathin section and freeze-fracture electron microscopy to study the surface characteristics and life cycle of *P. carinii* in steroid-treated rats (Yoneda et al., 1982). The following stages of the organism were noted: trophic or trophozoites (Figs. 11a and b); precysts (Figs. 12a and b); and cysts (Figs. 12a and b). Our findings suggested that the crescent-shaped cysts (Figs. 14a and b) were intermediate forms between precyst and cyst as suggested by Vossen et al. (1978) and not degenerative forms of the organism as suggested by others. The cell wall of the trophic stage showed membrane structures suggestive of protozoan endocytosis, whereas the surface of the precyst stage was smooth. The cell wall of the cyst stage lacked specialized structural differentiation of yeasts and resembled that of *Plasmodia.* On the basis of findings, we believe that *P. carinii* is a protozoan rather than a yeast.

IV. Experimental *P. carinii* Infection in Mice

In their studies of the effects of steroids on different animal species, Frenkel et al. (1966) found a mild *P. carinii* pneumonia in 1 of 4 autopsied mice. Since this work has not been pursued further, we undertook a study to determine whether the steroid-treated mouse could serve as a model for *P. carinii* infection (Walzer et al., 1979b).

The following strains of mice were used: C3H/HeN, C57BL/6N, BALB/cAnN, DBA/2N, B10.A(2R), DBA/1J, ARK/J, and outbred Swiss Webster mice. Female mice, all strains, weighing about 18-20 g were used. In some experiments male mice weighing 18-40 g were also used. Since a major object of the study was to find the optimal regimen for inducing pneumocystis pneumonia, a variety of dietary and corticosteroid doses were tried. The mice ate a regular or low protein diet ad libitum and drank tap water with or without tetracycline; in selected studies water intake was measured. Mice were weighed weekly. Corticosteroids were administered either as twice weekly subcutaneous injections of cortisone acetate or as dexamethasone added to the drinking water. The mice were sacrificed usually after 8-12 weeks, and lungs were processed as described previously for rats. Serum specimens were obtained by cardiac puncture and stored at -20°C. The intensity of *P. carinii* infection in lungs was assessed by the semiquantitative scoring system described above. In addition, the mean *P. carinii* score for each group of mice was calculated for the purpose of comparison; calculations were made only on those mice where *P. carinii* was seen (i.e., with a score of $\geq 0.5+$).

A considerable amount of trial-and-error was required to test different corticosteroid regimens. As seen in Figures 15a and b, a dose of 1 mg of cortisone acetate injected twice weekly combined with a low-protein diet produced moderate weight loss and was sufficient to produce demonstrable pneumocystis pneumonia. Doses of cortisone above 1 mg often shortened survival. Doses of dexamethasone in the drinking water equivalent to 1 mg of cortisone acetate were also successful in producing *P. carinii* pneumonia. The mice sometimes exhibited great variation in their sensitivity to the effects of corticosteroids. For example, BALB/cAnN mice obtained from one dealer tolerated a 2.5 mg dosage schedule of cortisone very well; yet the same strain obtained from another dealer and placed on the same regimen, started dying in great numbers within 2 weeks of beginning steroids. The cause of death in this and in other episodes of early fatalities appeared to be overwhelming bacterial infection. A variety of organisms were cultured, but there was not a single predominant pathogen. Thus, both steroid dose and pre-existing microbial flora appear to be important in determining the value of mice as experimental models for *P. carinii* infection.

The results of the study are seen in Table 1. For the purpose of analysis in this chapter the mice have been broadly categorized as "control" and "corticosteroid-treated," and the results for these categories have been pooled for each strain of mice. Control refers to nonsteroid-treated mice and includes various dietary regimens (e.g., regular and low-protein diet). Corticosteroid includes all steroid regimens. The original study should be consulted if there is interest in seeing the type of *P. carinii* pneumonia produced in a particular mouse strain with a particular corticosteroid regimen.

As can be seen in Table 1, *P. carinii* infection was found in a few control members of each mouse strain, with the exception of DBA/2N which had no *P. carinii* infection. Control mice remained healthy throughout the experiment, and the low *P. carinii* score of the infected mice is consistent with the subclinical carrier state in nature. Among steroid-treated mice, *P. carinii* was found in all strains. The intensity of the infection could be grouped into three broad categories: (1) C3H/HeN mice had the heaviest degree of infection; (2) BALB/cAnN, AKR/J, C57BL/6N, B10.A(2R), and Swiss Webster all had a high frequency but moderate intensity of the infection; and (3) DBA/2N and DBA/1J had both a lower frequency and a lower intensity of infection. The reasons for these differences in *P. carinii* infection are unclear. The survival of mice on corticosteroids was similar among the different strains except among DBA/1J mice where it was considerably shorter. The results suggest possible strain differences in susceptibility to *P. carinii* among the mice; however, this is difficult to prove because of the small numbers of mice used and the mechanism here is reactivation of latent infection rather than exogenous organism challenge.

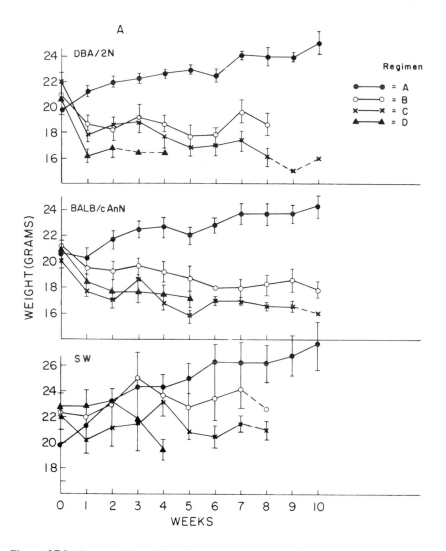

Figure 15A Sequential weight changes in mice in different corticosteroid regimens.   Each point represents the mean ± 1 SEM weight of at least 3 mice.   Dotted line indicates less than 3 mice in group.   Regimen A = controls; regimen B (1 mg), C (2:5 mg), and D (5 mg) are cortisone acetate doses injected subcutaneously twice weekly.   (From Walzer et al., 1979b.)

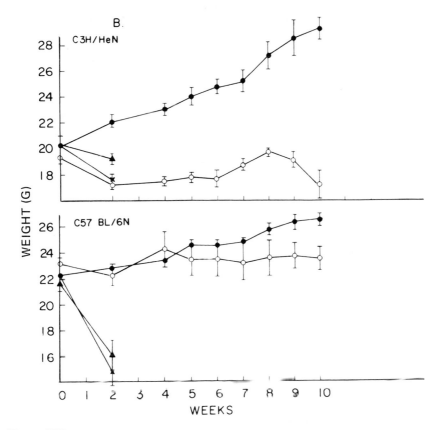

Figure 15B

Table 1 *Pneumocystis carinii* Infection in Different Strains of Normal Mice

Mouse strain	No. infected/total	Mean *P. carinii* score[a]
Corticosteroid		
C3H/HeN	27/30	1.9
BALB/cAnN	31/38	1.5
AKR/J	17/17	1.3
C57BL/6N	15/20	1.2
B10.A(2R)	10/14	1.1
Swiss Webster	13/16	1.1
DBA/2N	5/14	0.8
DBA/1J	4/17	0.8
Control		
C3H/HeN	2/12	0.5
BALB/cAnN	4/23	0.5
AKR/J	2/6	0.5
C57BL/6N	1/6	0.5
B10.A(2R)	1/6	0.5
Swiss Webster	1/9	0.5
DBA/2N	0/6	0.0
DBA/1J	2/7	0.5

[a]Calculated only where *P. carinii* was found (score ≥ 0.5).
Source: Walzer and Powell (1982).

The appearance of pneumocystis organisms on methenamine silver and Giemsa stains by light microscopy was morphologically indistinguishable from their rat or human counterparts. The histopathologic appearance of the host inflammatory responses was similar among the different strains of mice and resembled the features seen in the rat model. The major difference was that the intensity of the infection was generally less in mice than in the corticosteroid-treated rat; few mice obtained a 4+ *P. carinii* score. This may have been due to the fact that the optimal corticosteroid dose in mice (1 mg injected twice weekly or 14 mg/kg body weight per day) was slightly less than half the steroid dose used in rats (25 mg injected subcutaneously twice weekly or 30-35 mg/kg per day).

Thus, this study demonstrates that the corticosteroid-treated mouse can serve as an experimental model for pneumocystis pneumonia. Success of this model depends not only on the corticosteroid dose but also the strain, source, general health, and pre-existing microbial flora of the mice chosen for study.

V. Athymic (Nude) Mice

The nude mouse lacks a thymus gland, a trait inherited as an autosomal recessive trait. The nude mouse is unique because this "experiment of nature" provides a direct way to measure the role of cellular immunity in biologic phenomena or disease processes. Since its discovery, the nude mouse has gained widespread popularity as a powerful experimental tool in the fields of immunology, oncology, and infectious diseases (Fough and Giovenella, 1978).

At Memorial Sloan-Kettering Cancer Center (MSKCC) the author became interested in the nude mouse as a possible experimental model for *P. carinii* infection (Walzer et al., 1977). Outbred Swiss female nude (Nu/Nu) mice and haired (Nu/+) litter mates at least 5-weeks-old were used in the study; the mice were of an ICR background and were raised and maintained in an area of MSKCC apart from other animals. In the first series of experiments, intrapulmonary injection of *P. carinii* infected human or rat lung homogenates, either freshly obtained or frozen up to 3 months, resulted in *P. carinii* infection in a high proportion of nude mice (Table 2). Injection of lung homogenates frozen for longer periods of time and intranasal inoculation were largely unsuccessful. *Pneumocystis carinii* was absent among control nude mice raised apart from other animals, but was present in a few nude mice which had been placed in a room with corticosteroid-treated rats. In another series of experiments, *P. carinii* was introduced into the closed nude mouse colony. Over a period of 3 months, groups of nude mice were injected with lung homogenates from patients with pneumocystis pneumonia and were placed in the same cage with uninoculated nude mice; other nude mice occupying separate cages in the colony room were randomly selected as distant contact controls. As can be seen in Table 3, a high frequency of *P. carinii* infection was found in all groups of mice. A third group of experiments involved nude mice raised in isolators. These mice were divided into three groups. One group was placed in the same cage with corticosteroid-treated rats and separated by a metal screen to study the rat-to-mouse transmission of *P. carinii* by close contact. Two such cages were placed in a germ-free isolator. Another group of nude mice was placed in mouse cages on top of the special rat-mouse cages in the isolator to study the transmission by the airborne route. The third group of nude mice remained in the isolator colony. The experiment lasted 7 weeks, at which time the animals were sacrificed. As

Table 2 Transmission of Rat and Human *P. carinii* to Nude Mice by Inoculation of Infected Lung Homogenates

Method of inoculation	Lung homogenate		No. infected/total	Mean *P. carinii* score
	Source	Status		
Nu/Nu mice				
Intrapulmonary	Human	Fresh	8/10	1.8
Intrapulmonary	Human	Frozen	4/29	0.5
Intrapulmonary	Rat	Fresh	11/17	0.8
Intrapulmonary	Rat	Frozen	0/11	0.0
Intranasal	Human	Frozen	0/8	0.0
Intranasal	Rat	Fresh	0/8	0.0
Control[a]	-	-	0/84	0.0
Control[b]	-	-	6/39	0.8
Nu/+ mice				
Intrapulmonary	Human/rat	Fresh/frozen	1/20	0.5
Control[a]	-	-	0/10	0.0

[a]Remained in closed or isolator colonies.
[b]Housed in separate cages but same room with infected rats.
Source: Walzer et al. (1977) and Walzer and Powell (1982).

Table 3 Transmission of Human *P. carinii* Infection to Nude (Nu/Nu) Mice in a Closed Nude Mouse Colony

Mode of transmission	No. infected/total	Mean *P. carinii* score
Intrapulmonary injection of infected lung homogenates	9/21	1.0
Close contact[a]	7/10	1.2
Airborne (distant contact)[b]	16/23	1.7

[a]Mice occupying the same cages with injected mice.
[b]Mice occupying separate cages.
Source: Walzer et al. (1977) and Walzer and Powell (1982).

Table 4 Transmission of *P. carinii* Infection from Rats to Nude (Nu/Nu) Mice via the Environment

Mode of transmission	No. infected/total	Mean *P. carinii* score
Close contact[a]	9/10	1.1
Airborne[b]	6/10	0.8
Control[c]	0/18	0.0

[a]Mice occupying the same cage with corticosteroid-treated rats.
[b]Mice occupying separate cages placed on top of rat/mouse cages.
[c]Mice remaining in isolator colony.
Source: Walzer et al. (1977) and Walzer and Powell (1982).

can be seen in Table 4, *P. carinii* was found in both groups of nude mice exposed to the rats, but was absent in the controls. These studies demonstrated the environmental transmission of *P. carinii* by close contact. Airborne transmission was also suggested, but it was possible that small particles of infected matter (e.g., bedding) could have been transmitted to the mouse cages during cage changing.

Most nude mice infected with *P. carinii* did not appear clinically ill. The intensity of the infection was usually light and there was no difference in the distribution or appearance of rat and human organisms in the mouse lungs. On hematoxylin- and eosin-stained lung sections there was little host inflammatory response; indeed, it was difficult to distinguish infected from uninfected lungs by this stain.

These data suggest that the nude mouse might be a good potential experimental model for study of the epidemiologic features of *P. carinii* infection. These studies also represented the first instance where *P. carinii* from one species (man, rat) could be transmitted to another species. Because of this apparent communicability of *P. carinii,* studies with nude mice should be performed in isolators or other protected areas to avoid potential contamination from exogenous sources. While the nude mouse is of considerable interest, further manipulations will be necessary to increase the intensity of *P. carinii* infection achieved before the nude mouse can be used as a model to study the pathogenesis of *P. carinii* infection.

More recent studies performed at the Lexington VA Medical Center and University of Kentucky used an outbred Swiss nude mouse strain developed at the National Institutes of Health (NIH) (Walzer and Powell, 1982). These mice were obtained through an interagency agreement between the National Cancer Center of NIH and the Veterans' Administration. A breeding colony was established at the Lexington VA Medical Center, where Nu/Nu males were mated with Nu/+ females. The mice were housed in Bioclean units (Fieldstone Corp., Cincinnati, Ohio) in a room apart from other animals.

These studies were primarily designed to extend the results of the previous studies. Attention was devoted to such factors as establishing the incubation period of *P. carinii,* calculating inoculum size and minimal infective dosage, increasing the intensity of the infection, and developing new modes of transmission (e.g., aerosols). The first series of studies involved an attempt to transmit rat *P. carinii* into the nude mice by different methods of inoculation with infected rat lung homogenates. As seen in Table 5, these studies were largely unsuccessful. Specifically, the rate of *P. carinii* infection among inoculated animals was no higher than that observed in the controls. Among those animals where *P. carinii* was found, the infection was subclinical. These results occurred despite a variety of inoculation sizes and the maneuvers (e.g., corticosteroid administration), designed to increase the susceptibility of the mice to infection. In a second series of studies, attempts were made to transmit *P. carinii* from steroid-treated rats to the nude mice via the environment in germ-free isolators. The results of these studies (Table 6) were similar to those found in the first series of experiments. In a third series of studies, nude mice were placed in the same cage with corticosteroid-treated C3H/HeN mice but separated by a metal screen. The purpose was to investigate the transmission of mouse *P. carinii* by close contact. As seen in Table 7, a higher frequency of *P. carinii* infection was found in exposed mice than in control mice, suggesting that possible transmission of the organism occurred. The frequency of *P. carinii* was higher among exposed Nu/+ mice than among exposed Nu/Nu mice. It was unclear whether this represented a greater sensitivity of Nu/+ mice to mouse *P. carinii* or perhaps reflected the

Table 5 Transmission of Rat *P. carinii* Infection to Nude Mice by Different Methods of Inoculation

Method of inoculation	Dose range (no. cysts)	No. infected/total	Mean *P. carinii* score
Intrapulmonary	$5.4 \times 10^3 - 1.5 \times 10^6$		
Nu/Nu		5/80	0.5
Nu/Nu[a]		2/24	0.5
Nu/+		4/28	0.5
Intratracheal	$5.4 \times 10^3 - 7.8 \times 10^5$		
Nu/Nu		0/13	0.0
Nu/+		0/5	0.0
Intranasal	$5.4 \times 10^3 - 7.8 \times 10^5$		
Nu/Nu		0/9	0.0
Nu/+		-	-
Aerosol	$9.5 \times 10^5 - 7.9 \times 10^8$ [b]		
Nu/Nu		1/55	0.5
Nu/+		1/16	0.5
Control	-		
Nu/Nu		3/78	0.5
Nu/Nu[a]		0/18	0.0
Nu/+		0/28	0.0

[a] Received steroids.
[b] Per milliliter of homogenate.
Source: Walzer and Powell (1982).

longer survival (59 ± 4 days) for these mice than among Nu/Nu mice (40 ± 3 days).

The results of these studies performed in Kentucky with nude mice are in sharp contrast to studies performed at MSKCC in New York. The reasons for the differences are unclear, but a number of hypotheses can be offered. One is that there are strain or species differences in *P. carinii.* As indicated above, pneumocystis organisms found in a variety of animal species are morphologically indistinguishable, but previous attempts to transmit *P. carinii* from one animal species to another have failed (Farrow et al., 1972; Frenkel et al., 1966; Minielly et al., 1969). The rats used in our studies were adult

Table 6 Transmission of *P. carinii* Infection from Rats to Nude Mice via the Environment

Mode of transmission	No. infected/total	Mean *P. carinii* score
Airborne		
Nu/Nu	2/48	0.5
Nu/+	0/19	0.0
Close contact		
Nu/Nu	0/17	0.0
Nu/+	0/11	0.0
Control		
Nu/Nu	1/65	0.5
Nu/+	1/16	0.5

Source: Walzer and Powell (1982).

Table 7 Transmission of *P. carinii* Infection from Steroid-Treated C3H/HeN Mice to Nude Mice via the Environment

Mode of transmission	No. infected/total	Mean *P. carinii* score
Close contact		
Nu/Nu	4/23	0.5
Nu/+	6/14	0.6
Control		
Nu/Nu	1/18	0.5
Nu/+	0/13	0.0

Source: Walzer and Powell (1982).

Sprague-Dawley rats, but were obtained from different breeders and the studies were performed years apart; thus, it was impossible to determine whether strain species in rat *P. carinii* existed. However, the greater success achieved with the mouse *P. carinii* transmission experiments raises the possibility of some differences between rat and mouse organisms. This subject is again addressed in our studies of immunological characteristics of the organism.

Another possibility is that the results represent strain differences among the nude mice in susceptibility to *P. carinii.* Although the nude mice were outbred, they were of different genetic backgrounds. Our previous studies in corticosteroid-treated mice also raise the possibility of strain differences in susceptibility to *P. carinii*. This question will only be answered when the Nu/Nu trait is bred into different inbred strains. These animals can then be tested with exogenous *P. carinii* under identical experimental conditions.

A third possibility is that the results represent different environmental conditions. Environmental differences have influenced studies of immune function in nude mice. Nu/Nu mice can be more susceptible or more resistant than Nu/+ litter mates to infection, depending on a variety of factors, including per-existing microbial flora (Emmerling et al., 1975; Mogensen and Anderson, 1978). These factors contribute to the concept of "nonspecific resistance" in the nude mice, which is expressed, at least in part, by macro-phages; such resistance can be modified by antibiotic administration which alters the microbial flora (Hellstrom and Balish, 1979; Nickol and Bonventure, 1977). Nude mice in our earlier and later studies were raised in different environments, and it is impossible to assess this variable with any degree of accuracy. In future studies of *P. carinii* infection in different strains of nude mice, the mice must be raised in the same environment. In our experience, this variable can be best controlled by the investigator. Ideally, the nude mice should be raised and maintained at a single institution with well-defined microbial flora.

The only other studies of *P. carinii* in nude mice have come from Ueda et al. (1977) and Tamura and co-workers (Tamura et al., 1978), who found naturally occurring *P. carinii* pneumonia in a BALB/c nude mouse colony. Mice greater than 6 months old seemed to die from *P. carinii* infection, whereas mice 2-3 months old had lighter degrees of infection and did not appear to be clinically ill. The authors produced *P. carinii* infection in BALB/BALB/c Nu/+ mice by the administration of corticosteroids or cyclophospha-mide; infection was then transmitted by close contact to Nu/Nu mice in a manner similar to that in our studies.

We attempted to study *P. carinii* in BALB/cAnN nude mice obtained from the NCI-VA sharing agreement. Our efforts have been frustrated by lack of adequate numbers of mice, by the often poor state of health of the mice which were received, and by our inability to breed the mice at our in-stitution. In addition, we have also observed subclinical *P. carinii* infection among small members of BALB/c mice which appeared to have been present on arrival at our hospital.

VI. Other Experimental Animals

Over 20 years ago, Sheldon studied experimental *P. carinii* pneumonia in rab-bits (Sheldon, 1959b). As in the studies of Weller, he found *P. carinii* infection in corticosteroid-treated control rabbits. He concluded that the mechanism of the pneumonia produced was reactivation of latent infection. Histopathologically the pneumonia appeared quite similar to that observed in corticosteroid-treated rats and mice. There has been little other apparent interest in developing the rabbit as an experimental model.

Frenkel et al. (1966) administered corticosteroids to hamsters as part of their studies of the effects of these agents in different animals. Curiously, *P. carinii* infection was not found in the hamsters. Similar results have been found recently by Yoshida et al. (1981). The apparent resistance of hamsters to corticosteroid *P. carinii* pneumonia might provide some insight into the host factors of susceptibility or resistance to this organism.

A variety of cogenitally immunodeficient animals offer potential as animal models for *P. carinii* infection. The athymic (nude) rat (DeJong et al., 1980; Vos et al., 1980) is of particular interest because of the widespread experience with corticosteroid-treated rats. A number of different types of mice (e.g., asplenic mouse, CBA/N mouse, and motheaten streaker mouse) have been discovered (Lozzio, 1976; Scher et al., 1975; Shultz and Green, 1976) which may be helpful in the study of the host–parasite relationship with infectious agents. With modern breeding techniques, it should also be possible to combine some of these immune defects. Recently a nude or hairless guinea pig strain has been discovered, which so far has shown a short life span (Reed and O'Donoghue, 1982). One of the causes of death has been spontaneous pneumocystis pneumonia.

VII.   Purification of *P. carinii*

Investigative work with *P. carinii* has been hampered by the lack of a ready supply of large numbers of purified organisms. The author is envious of colleagues who can simply streak out a culture of bacteria or an agar plate and have untold numbers of organisms ready for use by the next morning! As described elsewhere (Chap. 5), modest success has been achieved with growing *P. carinii* in tissue culture (Bartlett et al., 1979; Latorre et al., 1977; Pifer et al., 1977, 1978a). A variety of tissue culture techniques have been used but were found to have the following limitations: (1) the degree of success with a particular technique in one laboratory has usually not been achieved in other laboratories and (2) long-term cultivation of *P. carinii* has not been accomplished. Thus, at present no one method of tissue culture has gained widespread use. Nevertheless, progress made in tissue culture has been encouraging, and hopefully improved techniques will be developed in the future.

Another approach has involved extraction of *P. carinii* from infected host tissues. The first step is usually a mechanical process in which small pieces of lung are ground with a tissue grinder, blender, mortar and pestle, etc. The second step involves enzymatic digestion. Some authors favor trypsin (Lim et al., 1973, 1974), while others prefer collagenase (Hendley and Weller, 1971; Ikai et al., 1977) or pronase (Meuwissen et al., 1973). N-acetyl-L-cysteine has been advocated when tracheobronchial washings have been the source of *Pneumocystis* organisms (Kim et al., 1972). Some authors have not used enzymes, but have advocated crude fractional centrifugation (Minielly et al., 1970; Norman and Kagan, 1970) or freezing and thawing procedures (Ikai, 1980). In the final step of this process some investigators have used sucrose density gradient centrifugation (Lim et al., 1973; Norman and Kagan, 1970) while others have relied on passage of contents through filters of different pore sizes (Ikai et al., 1977; Meuwissen et al., 1973).

We developed a new separation technique which was patterned after separation of lymphocytes from hematopoietic and lymphoid organs (Walzer et al., 1979a). In the first step, lung tissue was cut up into pieces and homogenized with a Teflon pestle and no. 60 wire mesh screen; this resulted in a more even suspension of organisms without visible chunks of host tissue. The second step involved digestion with a variety of enzymes. The lung homogenate was incubated with the enzyme to be tested at a variety of different enzyme concentrations and for different periods of time. Pronase at concentrations of 0.05 and 0.25% virtually destroyed *P. carinii;* trypsin seemed to produce some morphologic alterations in *P. carinii* on CEV stain and did not completely digest the lung tissue. These enzymes have been studied in detail in a separate report (Stahr et al., 1981) which will be discussed below. Papain and N-acetyl-L-cysteine also did not adequately digest lung tissue. By contrast, collagenase digested the lung tissue well and left *P. carinii* intact; this effect was enhanced by the addition of hyaluronidase, and thus these two enzymes became part of the working solution for routine digestion of lung tissue. The optimal concentration of each enzyme was 0.2%. In the third step, we employed a 10-layer discontinuous gradient composed of Ficoll and Hypaque solutions. The lung homogenate was applied to the gradient and centrifuged at 600 g for 30 min at room temperature. Initial studies were performed with rat *P. carinii.* Layer 1 was an enriched trophozoite layer. Layer 2 contained a mixture of cysts and trophozoites. Layers 3 and 4 were an enriched cyst layer (Fig. 16), although clumps of trophozoites could be found. Layers 5-7 had clumps of *P. carinii* and pieces of host tissue, whereas in layers 8-10 there were even larger pieces of tissue and debris.

The Ficoll-Hypaque gradient has proven a useful separation technique. It has produced no light or electron microscopic alterations in *P. carinii,* but its effects on organism viability are unknown. The wash solution in the gradient is Hanks' balanced salt solution without calcium or magnesium, but containing 1 mM ethylene diaminetetraacetate (EDTA). This solution appeared

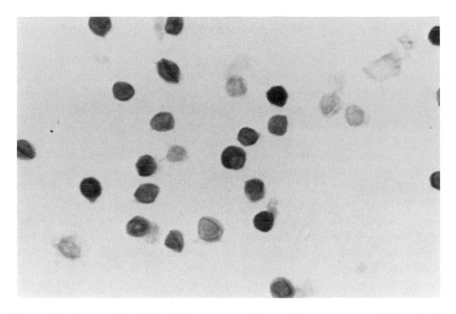

Figure 16 Layer 3-4 of Ficoll-Hypaque gradient. *P. carinii* cysts with typical morphology are seen. (Cresyl echt violet, ×1250.) (From Walzer et al., 1979a.)

to enhance the digestive activities of the enzyme and also helped prevent clumping of organisms. The Ficoll-Hypaque gradient has also been applied to human and mouse infected lungs. Human organisms tended to clump more than did rat organisms and human *P. carinii* cysts were best found in layers 3-6. Several mouse lungs have to be pooled to obtain enough organisms to be applied to the gradient. Our work with mouse *P. carinii* has primarily involved immunoflourescent studies and we have used organisms derived from layers 1-6 or the gradient.

VIII. Immunologic Studies

We have conducted a series of immunologic studies of rat, human, and mouse *P. carinii* (Milder et al., 1980; Stahr ct al., 1981; Walzer and Rutledge, 1980, 1981, 1982). These studies have involved evaluation of the antigenic characteristics of the organism, measurement of serum antibodies to *P. carinii,* and application of immunologic techniques for the clinical diagnosis of pneumocystis pneumonia. The major immunologic technique has been the indirect flourescent antibody (IFA) technique.

In the first series of experiments antisera were raised to rat *P. carinii* in rabbits (Milder et al., 1980). The following organism preparations were used: (1) enriched cyst or trophozoite layers of whole organisms derived from Ficoll-Hypaque gradients; (2) Ficoll-Hypaque gradient-enriched cyst fractions which were sonicated or treated with hydrochloric acid; and (3) bronchial lavage fluid specimens which had been lyophilized. The rabbits were immunized with a series of subcutaneous injections of *P. carinii* in normal saline first mixed with complete and then incomplete Freund's adjuvant. Some rabbits received a series of intravenous injections of whole *Pneumocystis* organisms alone or following subcutaneous injections. The rabbits were bled at appropriate intervals; the serum specimens were absorbed first with rat liver powder or uninfected rat lung and then with serum from uninfected rats.

The rabbit sera were tested for antibodies to *P. carinii* by the IFA technique. First, 5 μl of Ficoll-Hypaque layers 2 or 3-4 were placed in each of 8 wells of clean Teflon-coated glass slides and were heat fixed. Serial dilutions (25 μl) of the serum to be tested were added to the wells; the slide was incubated in a moist chamber at 37°C for 45 min and was washed twice with phosphate-buffered saline (PBS), pH 7.2-7.4. Next, 25 μl of flourescein-conjugated goat anti-rabbit IgG (Cappel Labs, Cochranville, PA) at an appropriate dilution was added to each well; the slide was incubated and washed as above. The slide was then mounted in glycerin-PBS and read with a Leitz Orthoplan flourescence microscope. The intensity of the fluorescence was graded on a scale from 0 (negative) to 4+ (maximum). The highest dilution with a 1+ intensity of flourescence was considered to be the peak antibody titer. As seen in Table 8, antibody titers were achieved with a variety of *P. carinii* preparations. Whole organisms injected subcutaneously and/or intravenously gave the highest antibody titers. No antibodies were obtained with rabbits immunized with lung homogenates from germ-free rats. No cross reactions were obtained with a variety of bacteria and fungi. From these and other tests, the antisera appeared specific for *P. carinii*.

Pneumocystis organisms derived from the Ficoll-Hypaque gradients stained brightly with a typical rim pattern of flourescence (Fig. 17a). Organisms from lung imprint smears were morphologically indistinguishable by IFA. Bronchial lavage fluids from infected animals were centrifuged, 5 μl of sediment were placed in the well of the Teflon-coated glass slide, and the IFA test was performed; the organisms which flouresced were identical to those above (Fig. 17b). Thus, at least by the IFA technique, digestion with collagenase and hyaluronidase and centrifugation on Ficoll-Hypaque density gradient did not alter the immunogenicity of *P. carinii*.

Table 8 Rabbit Antisera to *P. carinii*

Rabbit	Immunogen source	No. cysts	Route	Reciprocal peak IFA titer
1, 2	FHL_{3-4}[a]	$7.1 \times 10^6 - 2.5 \times 10^7$	s.c.	128
3, 4	FHL_{3-4}	$7.0 \times 10^5 - 2.5 \times 10^7$	s.c/i.v.	512
5	FHL_{3-4}	$7.0 \times 10^5 - 2.8 \times 10^6$	i.v.	256
6	FHL_{3-4}	HCl extract (1.6×10^7)	s.c.	4
7	FHL_{3-4}	Sonicated (3.3×10^7)	s.c.	32
8	FHL_2	2.8×10^5	s.c.	256
9	FHL_2	$2.0 \times 10^5 - 2.0 \times 10^6$	i.v.	256
10	FHL_1	1.1×10^5	s.c.	64
11, 12, 13	Bronchial lavage fluid	Lyophilized ($1.2 \times 10^5 - 6.2 \times 10^5$)	s.c.	16
14	Germ-free rat	Lung homogenate (none)	s.c.	0

[a]FHL = Ficoll-Hypaque layer.
Source: Milder et al. (1980).

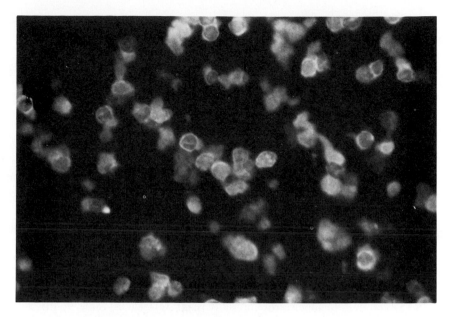

Figure 17a Immunofluorescent staining of *P. carinii*. The organisms stain brightly in a typical peripheral rim pattern. Here is *P. carinii* isolated from a Ficoll-Hypaque gradient (×1250). (From Milder et al., 1980.)

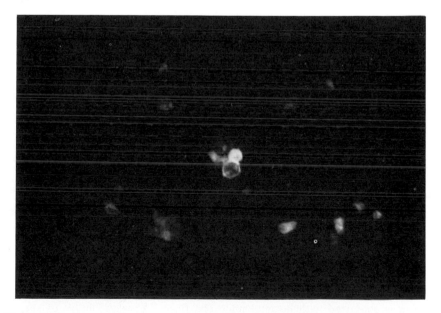

Figure 17b *P. carinii* in bronchial lavage fluid (×1250). (From Milder et al., 1980.)

A study was then performed comparing morphological and immunological techniques in the early detection of *P. carinii* in the bronchial lavage
fluid of steroid-treated rats. Preliminary experiments indicated that a semiquantitative assessment of the intensity of *P. carinii* infection in bronchial
lavage fluid based on detection of cysts by CEV stain correlated well with
previously described semiquantitative assessment in rat lung parenchyma.
Members of rat groups A, B, and C used in the previous study of *P. carinii*
infection were used here; since *P. carinii* infection developed in all rats
treated with steroids beyond two weeks, group B and C rats have been combined here for the purpose of analysis. In the protocol, 2–4 rats were sacrificed weekly for 11 weeks; lung specimens for histologic examination and
bronchial lavage fluid were obtained for each rat. The technique of bronchial lavage and the method of preparing the sediment have been described
in detail elsewhere (Milder et al., 1980). Lavage fluid sediments were then
examined for the presence of *P. carinii* using the following techniques: (1)
CEV stain, (2) Giemsa stain, (3) IFA techniques, (4) double diffusion (DD),
and (5) counterimmunoelectrophoresis (CIE). As seen in Table 9, the results
showed that CEV detected *P. carinii* as early as the second week of steroid
treatment, and in all specimens after that. Giemsa stain did not detect the
organism until 4 weeks; the organism disappeared with steroid tapering at
weeks 10 and 11. The organism was detected with IFA as early as 1 week
and in all specimens at $\geq$ 3 weeks. The organism could not be detected by
DD or CIE.

Several conclusions can be drawn from this study. First, a selective
cell wall stain, such as CEV, appears to be more sensitive in detecting *P.
carinii* then does the Giemsa stain. As in studies of quantitation, the Giemsa
stain stains a variety of host tissue cells, thus making it difficult to identify
the organism with certainty. This is not to imply that persons who have a
special interest or expertise in Giemsa stain could not identify *P. carinii* more
readily than was done in this study. However, cell wall stains are much more
widely used in routine clinical labs; thus, if the results in our rat model can
be extrapolated to patients, cell wall stains, in the author's opinion, are preferable in the diagnosis of *P. carinii* infection.

Secondly, immunoflourescence is a sensitive and specific method of detecting *P. carinii* in tissue specimens. Larger numbers of animals would have
to be sampled to accurately compare IFA with CEV stains. One area where
IFA might have value is when very few organisms are present; here *P. carinii*
can be confused with yeasts and the availability of a specific antibody might
be helpful in the differentiation. Our rats were also colonized in their lavage
fluid with a variety of bacteria, particularly *Flavobacterium meningosepticum.*
Again, these rats might have some relevance to the seriously ill patient who
becomes colonized with hospital microbial flora. The availability of specific

Table 9 Techniques Detecting *P. carinii* Infection

No. positive specimens/no. examined

| | Weeks | | | | | | | | | | | |
Technique	0	1	2	3	4	5	6	7	8	9	10	11
Lungs												
Histology	1/3	2/3	3/3	3/3	4/4	4/4	4/4	4/4	3/3	3/3	2/2	1/1
Bronchial lavage fluid												
Cresyl violet	0/3	0/3	2/3	3/3	4/4	4/4	4/4	4/4	3/3	3/3	2/2	1/1
Giemsa	0/3	0/3	0/3	0/3	3/4	4/4	3/4	3/4	2/3	2/3	0/2	0/1
IFA	0/3	1/3	2/3	3/3	4/4	4/4	4/4	4/4	3/3	3/3	2/2	1/1
DD/CIE	0/3	0/3	0/3	0/3	0/4	0/4	0/4	0/4	0/3	0/3	0/2	0/1

Source: Milder et al. (1980).

antiserum to identify *P. carinii* may also be helpful in this patient population.

A recent study has shown that most children with pneumocystis pneumonia have soluble *P. carinii* antigen in their serum, detectable by CIE (Pifer et al., 1978b). This finding is of considerable potential importance because it would provide a rapid noninvasive method of diagnosing *P. carinii* infection. However, in another study (Meyers et al., 1979), these investigators noted a high frequency of circulating antigen in patients without tissue evidence of *P. carinii*, thus raising questions about the specificity of the test. Further studies are needed to determine whether the antigen being detected is truly derived from *P. carinii* or perhaps represents some lung-associated component.

Despite a variety of experimental maneuvers detailed elsewhere (Milder et al., 1980), we were unable to raise specific precipitating antibodies to *P. carinii* or to find soluble *P. carinii* antigens in the serum or lavage fluid of our rats.

Further studies are needed to improve the diagnosis of *P. carinii* infection by immunological techniques. Bronchial lavage offers advantages over simple bronchoscopy with washings becasue large volumes of alveolar effluent can be sampled with low morbidity from the procedure. Bronchial alveolar lavage has been used to diagnose pneumocystis pneumonia by histologic techniques (Kelley et al., 1978), and might provide an ideal medium to detect *P. carinii* antigens if a sensitive technique (e.g., radioimmunoassay, enzyme-linked immunosorbent assay, etc.) could be developed. Efforts to detect these antigens in serum and perhaps even in urine should continue. The corticosteroid-treated rat provides an excellent model to develop these techniques.

In another study (Stahr et al., 1981), we compared the effects of digestion with trypsin and pronase on *P. carinii* in infected rat lung homogenates. Since *P. carinii* trophozoites were markedly reduced in number by enzyme digestion, our attention was devoted to the cysts. Enzymes were compared at different concentrations and at different times of exposure. Cysts digested with trypsin at concentrations of 0.1-1.0% exhibited swelling of their cell wall as seen by electron microscopy; these changes could also be seen on light microscopy by CEV and Giemsa stains. Pronase at concentrations of 0.01-0.25% caused a reduction in the number of cysts; the major morphological change in the cysts was loss of the cell wall. The effects of these enzymes were also compared by IFA. Rat lung homogenates were placed in wells of the Teflon-coated slide, serial dilutions of rabbit antiserum to *P. carinii* were added, and the IFA test was performed. *P. carinii* cysts digested with trypsin stained brightly in a manner similar to that of control cysts. The peak antiserum titer was 1:512 in both trypsin-digested and control cysts. On the other hand, pronase digestion produced dose-related changes in the antiserum titer by IFA. At a pronase concentration of 0.01%, the IFA titer was 1:256 at both 1 and 5 min of enzyme exposure, but fell to 1:16 at 30 min of exposure. No fluorescent staining occurred at enzyme concentrations of 0.05, 0.1, and 0.25%.

We concluded from this study that trypsin and pronase have different actions on *P. carinii* cysts. The actions of trypsin are directed toward the positively charged side chains with arginine and lysine (Decker, 1977). The enzymatic activity of pronase is broader and includes activity against certain structural components (e.g., N-acetylhexosamine, sialic acid) and neutral sugars (e.g., galactose) (Hashimoto et al., 1963). This study also demonstrates how enzymes can reveal certain characteristics of *P. carinii*. The data suggest that the antigenic determinants of *P. carinii* cysts reside in the cell wall.

Enzyme digestion has revealed important information about the surface characteristics of other organisms. A good example of this can be seen in the studies of receptor sites on host cells for the attachment of *Mycoplasma pneumoniae* in organ culture systems (Gabridge and Taylor-Robinson, 1979). These methods might also be applicable to the study of *P. carinii* trophozoites in terms of their attachment to host alveolar type 1 cells. Moreover, the use of such techniques as immunoferritin or immunoperoxidase staining, when combined with electron microscopy, might also help in localizing the antigen-combining sites of the organism.

As detailed in Chap. 4, IFA, and to a lesser extent, complement fixation, have been the principal methods for measuring serum antibodies to *P. carinii*. Serology has been helpful in the clinical diagnosis of pneumocystis pneumonia in institutionalized infants with the epidemic form of disease (Barta, 1969; Brzosko et al., 1967; Dutz, 1970; Meuwissen and Leeuwenberg, 1972), but has been of little help in the diagnosis of *P. carinii* in immunosuppressed patients (Lim et al., 1974; Meuwissen et al., 1977; Meyers et al., 1979; Norman and Kagan, 1973; Pifer et al., 1978b, Shepherd et al., 1979). Since serum antibodies occur in about 5-10% of close contacts of *P. carinii* patients, but are rare in the general population, serology found some use of the epidemiologic investigation of hospital outbreaks of pneumocystis pneumonia (Perera et al., 1970; Ruebush et al., 1978; Singer et al., 1975). More recent IFA studies suggest that about 75% of these patients develop serum antibodies to *P. carinii* by about 4 years of age (Meuwissen et al., 1977; Pifer et al., 1978b). The striking differences in these studies compared with earlier ones probably reflect differences in antigen preparations and criteria for determining an IFA-positive test. These studies emphasize the need for uniform standards in the IFA technique for *P. carinii* and, perhaps more importantly, a need for development of new serological techniques.

The source of antigens and antisera has been an important determining factor in the use of immunofluorescence in the study of *P. carinii.* Procedures used to purify *P. carinii* have included mechanical separation techniques and in vitro cultivation outlined previously. Sources of antisera have included animals immunized with *P. carinii* or serum specimens from humans or animals recovering from pneumocystis pneumonia. Both the IFA and direct flourescent antibody (DFA) techniques have been used. Some studies have demonstrated cross reactivity between rat and human *P. carinii* with antisera raised in rabbits (Ikai, 1980; Lim et al., 1973). In other studies, rat *P. carinii* has been substituted for human *P. carinii* to measure serum antibodies to the organism in patients (Gentry et al., 1972; Lim et al., 1974; Norman and Kagan, 1973). By contrast, studies of rats immunized with rat *P. carinii* obtained by bronchial lavage have shown no cross reactivity between rat and human *P. carinii* in lungs by IFA (Kim et al., 1972).

In our recent study (Walzer and Rutledge, 1980) we compared the antigenic characteristics of rat, mouse, and human *P. carinii* of the IFA technique. *Pneumocystis* organisms were separated from infected rat, human, and mouse lungs by Ficoll-Hypaque density gradient centrifugation. Antisera to rat and human *P. carinii* were produced in rabbits by injection of whole organisms as previously described. These antisera were then reacted against purified rat, human, or mouse *P. carinii* by the IFA technique. Prior to testing, rabbit antiserum to rat *P. carinii* was first absorbed with rat liver powder and then with rat, mouse, or human serum (depending upon which source of *P. carinii* was being tested) to further ensure specificity. Similar absorptions were performed with the rabbit antiserum to human *P. carinii.* As seen in Table 10, both antisera reacted to all three sources of *P. carinii,* suggesting shared antigenic determinant. Highest antibody titers were found with the homologous source of *P. carinii,* thus suggesting a degree of host specificity.

Pneumocystis organisms in tissue specimens stained brightly by IFA both antisera. Figure 18 shows a lung imprint smear of human *P. carinii* which reacted with antiserum to rat *P. carinii.* The organisms were morphologically indistinguishable when antiserum to human *P. carinii* was substituted. Similar results were obtained with mouse and rat lung imprint smears.

Serum antibodies in rats, mice, and humans were then tested against rat, mouse, and human sources of *P. carinii.* As seen in the Table 10, serum specimens from 6 rats with high antibody titers to rat *P. carinii* also had good antibody titers to mouse *P. carinii*; however, only 3 serum specimens reacted with human *P. carinii,* all in titers of 1:4. Serum specimens from 6 mice with high antibody titers to mouse *P. carinii* showed little or no reactivity to rat or human *P. carinii.* Four of 6 serum specimens from humans showed some reactivity to rat and mouse *P. carinii.* In 3 of these cases, the titer was only 1:4. The person with titer of 1:8 had worked in the *P. carinii*-infected rat and mouse colonies for more than one year.

Table 10 Serum Antibody Titers to Rat, Mouse, and Human *P. carinii* Among Different Animal Species

Animal species	Number of specimens	Range of reciprocal IFA titer		
		Source of *P. carinii*		
		Rat	Mouse	Human
Rat	6	64-1024 (6)[a]	128-512 (6)	4-4 (3)
Mouse	6	0-4 (2)	64-256 (6)	0 (0)
Human	6	0-8 (4)	0-8 (4)	16-128 (6)
Rabbit A[b]	1	512	32	8
Rabbit B[c]	1	32	32	512

[a]Numbers in parentheses indicate number of specimens with positive titer (i.e., ≥ 4).
[b]Immunized with rat *P. carinii*.
[c]Immunized with human *P. carinii*.
Source: Walzer and Rutledge (1980).

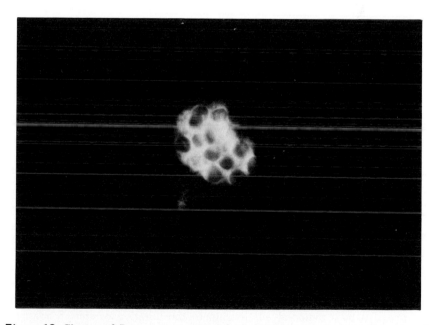

Figure 18 Cluster of *P. carinii* organisms from human lung, immunofluorescent staining, ×1250.

This study showed the advantage of using more than one source of antibody when comparing the antigenic properties of *P. carinii* derived from different animal species. By quantitating the antibody titer, the study also allowed the assessment of the degree of cross reactivity. Overall in our study, mouse and rat *P. carinii* appeared more closely related antigenically to each other than to human *P. carinii.* These data and results of transmission experiments by us and by other investigators support the hypothesis that there are strain or species differences in *P. carinii.*

An unresolved issue is whether there are antigenic differences in the different stages of the life cycle (e.g., cyst, trophozoite) of *P. carinii.* Some authors have noted such differences (Ikai, 1980; Lim et al., 1971), but in most studies this question has not been addressed in any detail. We have not noted differences between *P. carinii* cysts and trophozoites in our IFA studies. For example, trophozoites stain brightly with antisera made to enriched cyst fractions of Ficoll-Hypaque gradients and vice versa. However, our attention has focused more on the cyst because this form is easier to identify when determining the titer of an antiserum. On electron microscopy we have found the deposition of certain stains (e.g., periodic acid-silver) in the cell wall of cysts and intracellularly in trophozoites (Yoneda and Walzer, 1980). This suggests that certain cell wall constituents are synthesized or stored at different locations in the maturation process from trophozoite to cyst, and raises the possibility of antigenic differences in the cell surfaces of different stages of *P. carinii.*

There is little data available on the prevalence of serum antibodies to *P. carinii* among various animal populations. In two studies, small numbers of rats developed antibodies by IFA and immunodiffusion 6-8 weeks after steroids had been abruptly terminated (Frenkel et al., 1966; Lim et al., 1971). We began some studies to investigate the humoral immune responses to *P. carinii* infection in rats and mice (Walzer and Rutledge, 1981, 1982). The specimens used were largely obtained from the animals used in our early studies.

In our initial study, rats were divided into group A (controls), group B (steroid-treated), and group C (steroid-tapered) rats as described previously. The rats were sacrificed at weekly intervals and serum antibodies to rat *P. carinii* were measured by IFA. As seen in Figure 19, serum antibody titers varied among the three groups of rats, but certain patterns emerged. Most of the group A rats sacrificed at the beginning of this study had antibody titers of $\leqslant$ 1:4, but all rats from this group sacrificed at 10-12 weeks had titers of $\geqslant$ 1:16. About 50% of the group B rats on the standard steroid treatment regimen failed to develop antibody titers throughout the experiment. The remaining rats had antibody titers usually $\leqslant$ 1:64, but there did not appear to be a temporal relationship to the duration of steroid adminis-

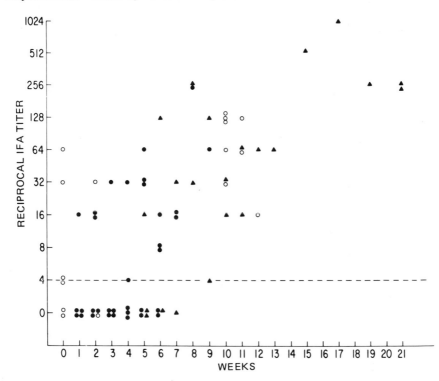

Figure 19 Sequential changes in rat serum antibody titers to *P. carinii* by IFA technique over time. ○, Group A controls; ●, group B rats in the standard corticosteroid regimen; ▲, group C rats, whose corticosteroid dose had been tapered. (From Walzer and Rutledge, 1982).

tration. Group C rats showed a progressive rise in antibody titers over time, with peak titers being obtained at ≥ 15 weeks.

In another experiment, 49 young (3-week-old) rats weighing about 50 g were obtained from a single dealer. The rats were placed in standard cages, ate a regular diet, drank tap water without tetracycline, and received no steroids. The rats were housed in the conventional rat colony room, which also housed steroid-treated rats. The rats were sacrificed every 1-2 weeks for 21 weeks. No serum antibodies to *P. carinii* were present in the rats for the first 8 weeks. Beginning at 10 weeks, the rats exhibited a progressive rise in serum antibody titers to the organism over time.

In a third experiment, 6 adult rats weighing approximately 200 g each were obtained from five different commercial laboratories. In addition, 6 retired breeder male rats about 6 months old and weighing about 500 g were obtained from two of these breeders. All rats were sacrificed upon arrival at the Lexington VAMC animal facility. The 30 young healthy adult rats contained no serum antibodies to *P. carinii*. However, all 12 retired breeder rats had serum antibody titers of $\geq$ 1:16.

In a fourth experiment, 8 young (3-week-old) rats obtained from a single commercial laboratory were bled via tail vein upon arrival at the Lexington VAMC. The rats were housed in the conventional rat colony room, where they ate a regular diet, drank tap water without tetracycline, and received no corticosteroids. After 3 weeks on this regimen, the rats were randomly divided into groups A, B, and C as described above. The object of the study was to measure sequential serum specimens in the same rat; thus, tail vein bleedings were obtained from the rats every 3-6 weeks. The study was terminated at 18 weeks. None of the group A control rats exhibited serum antibodies for the first 12 weeks, but by 18 weeks, all of these rats had developed serum antibody titers to the organism. None of the group B rats exhibited serum antibody titers throughout the study period. Group C rats developed serum antibodies by 18 weeks, and the titers were higher than those in group A rats.

These experiments demonstrate that young healthy adult rats do not usually have serum antibodies to *P. carinii*. Administration of corticosteroids and a low-protein diet to produce heavy *P. carinii* infection impaired antibody formation of the organism. With corticosteroid tapering and restoration of normal immune function, the animals developed high antibody titers to the organism. The experiments also demonstrate that the host develops serum antibodies to *P. carinii* with prolonged environmental exposure; this was found in rats housed in the rat colony room and in older rats obtained from commercial laboratories. Thus, these experiments support the studies in humans which show an increasing frequency of serum antibody titers to *P. carinii* with age (Meuwissen et al., 1977; Pifer et al., 1978b). The serum antibodies measured by IFA in the rats were of the IgG class. Flourescein-conjugated heavy-chain-specific antiserum to rat IgM and IgA are unavailable commercially; thus studies of these antibody classes were not performed.

We also measured quantitative immunoglobulin levels in rat serum specimens. IgG levels were determined in a commercially prepared kit. Antisera ti IgA and IgM were available from Miles Laboratories (Marion, IN) and we absorbed these with rat IgG in an attempt to enhance specificity. Immunoglobulin levels in rats have been measured by other investigators (Bazin et al., 1974; McGhee et al., 1975), but uniform standards are not yet available. We attempted to create standards by using pooled normal rat serum and applying the values of other investigators. While not completely satisfactory, this technique sufficed to measure relative changes in the immunoglobulin levels over time in *P. carinii* infection. In the first experiment, serum immunoglobulins were measured in group A, B, and C rats sacrificed at weekly intervals as described above. As seen in Figure 20, mean serum

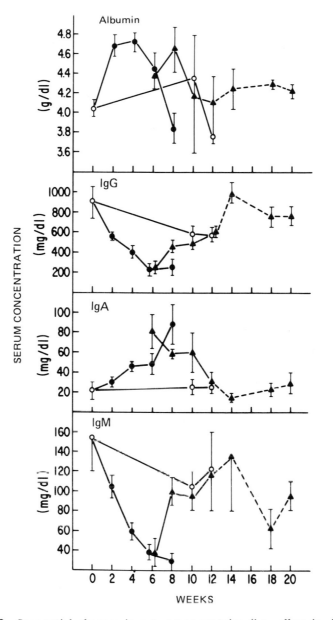

Figure 20 Sequential changes in rat serum proteins (i.e., albumin, IgG, IgA, or IgM) levels over time. Each point on the solid line represents the mean ± 1 SEM protein concentration of at least 3 rats. Dotted line represents less than 3 rats in the group. ○, Group A; ●, group B; ▲, group C rats as in Figure 33. (From Walzer and Rutledge, 1982.)

IgG and IgM levels declined markedly in group B rats but increased in group C rats after steroids had been discontinued. Mean serum IgA levels rose in group B rats and fell in group C rats, whereas the serum levels of all immunoglobulins in group A rats were largely unchanged. Serum albumin levels initially rose and then fell in group B rats, but no definitive pattern could be seen in group A or C rats. In the second study, where serial bleedings were performed in the same rats, serum levels of all immunoglobulins were considerably lower than in the first study. This probably reflected the younger age of the rats here. The patterns of change of immunoglobulins in groups A, B, and C of this study were similar to those observed in the first study.

Attention then focused on bronchial lavage fluid. As indicated previously, when lavage fluid was centrifuged, *Pneumocystis* organisms were present in the sediment. The supernatant was then concentrated by ultrafiltration in a uniform manner and then was tested for antibodies to *P. carinii* by IFA. The levels of albumin, IgG, IgM, and IgA were also measured in these concentrated lavage supernatants. The rats used here were group A, B, and C rats described above.

Antibody titers measured in lavage fluid of 55 rats correlated well with those obtained in serum (P < 0.001). Lavage fluid antibody levels were usually lower than serum antibody levels; in 11 rats, the lavage fluid titer equaled or exceeded its serum counterpart (Fig. 21). Highest lavage fluid antibody titers in groups A, B, or C rats tended to occur late in the course of the study. Albumin was found in all lavage fluids where it was measured, and the levels in lavage fluid were only 8-15% of serum levels (Table 11). IgA was found in 38% of lavage fluids tested and levels in lavage fluid varied widely when compared with serum levels. IgG and IgM were not detected in lavage fluids.

A number of authors have felt that since albumin is not synthesized in the lung the ratio of levels of albumin in bronchial lavage fluid to serum can be used as a standard of whether the presence of a substance in lavage fluid represents local production or merely passage from serum into lavage fluid (Hunninghake et al., 1979). Antibody titers to *P. carinii* in lavage fluid often exceeded 15% of serum antibody titers, thus, suggesting that at least a portion of the bronchial lavage fluid antibodies were locally produced. There is little available data on quantitative levels of immunoglobulins in rat bronchial lavage fluid.

We also conducted an experiment to determine whether immunoglobulins were on the surface of *P. carinii* in bronchial lavage fluid sediments. We used the DFA technique for rat IgG. We modified the IFA technique for IgA and IgM and also used a DFA technique with antisera to mouse IgA and IgM. We studied lavage fluid sediments from 30 group B and C rats after

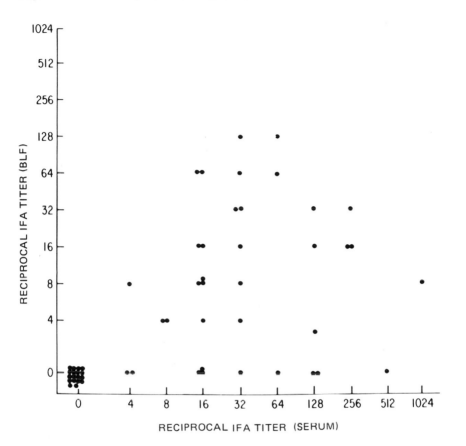

Figure 21 Antibody titers to *P. carinii* in serum (horizontal axis) and bronchial lavage fluid (vertical axis). Each point represents a single rat. (From Walzer and Rutledge, 1982.)

≥ 2 weeks of corticosteroid administration. We found IgG, IgA, and IgM on the surface of *P. carinii* in all lavage fluid sediments. The pattern of flourescent staining was similar to that obtained with specific antiserum to *P. carinii*. We had partial success in eluting IgG from the surface of the organism by incubation in acid citrate buffer, pH 3.2.

The detection of IgG, IgM, and IgA on the surface of *P. carinii* in bronchial lavage fluid sediments suggests that more than one immunoglobulin class is involved in the host immune response to the infection. Brzosko, et al., (1971) found IgG, IgM, and trace amounts of IgA on the surface of *P. carinii* in alveolar of lung sections of patients with pneumocystis pneumonia.

Table 11 Proteins Detected in Bronchial Lavage Fluid of Rats

Protein	No. detected/total	Range of values	% Of serum values (range)
Albumin	31/31	0.37-0.71 g/dl	8-15%
IgA	21/55	4-80 mg/dl	11-98%
IgG	0/55	-	-
IgM	0/55	-	-

Source: Walzer and Rutledge (1981).

It is possible that immunoglobulins function as opsonins and this has been discussed in Chapter 3. Recent studies have suggested that antibody does not alter the viability of *P. carinii* in vitro (Pesanti, 1980).

In a separate study we determined the serum antibody titers to *P. carinii* in mice (Walzer and Rutledge, 1982). The mice were part of studies of experimental *P. carinii* infection which have been described previously. In most cases mouse *P. carinii* was the antigen used, but in some instances (particularly with nude mice) rat *P. carinii* was also used. Standard IFA was performed. The major addition was the fact that antibody titers of IgG, IgM, and IgA classes were determined.

With normal mice 53 (73%) of 73 mouse sera tested had serum antibodies to mouse *P. carinii* present with at least one of the immunoglobulin classes (Table 12). Serum antibodies of more than one immunoglobulin class were found in 28 (54%) of the 53 mouse sera. These antibodies were mainly IgG and IgM. Only 16 (30%) of the mice had serum antibodies of the IgG class only, and 9 (17%) mice had antibodies only of the IgM class.

Serum antibodies to *P. carinii* were found in 5 of 6 strains of mice tested. Among C3H/HeN mice, the serum antibodies were found in all 5 control mice and in 6 of 10 steroid-treated mice. IgG was the major immunoglobulin class of antibody in both groups of mice; IgM antibodies were less frequent and IgA antibodies were very rare. Among BALB/cAnN mice, serum antibodies were predominantly of the IgG class; titers among control mice were higher than in steroid-treated mice. IgG was also the predominant class of antibody found among AKR/J and B10.A(2R) mice. By contrast, IgM antibodies were the predominant immunoglobulin class detected among steroid-treated C57BL/6N mice. No antibodies were found among DBA/1J mice, but the survival times of these mice were shorter than those of other groups of mice; steroid-treated DBA/1J mice were not tested.

In another study, BALB/cAnN mice were divided into group A (control)

Table 12 Serum Antibodies to *P. Carinii* in Different Strains of Normal Mice

Mouse strain	Survival (days)[a]	No. seropositive[b]/total
Corticosteroid-treated		
C3H/HeN	62±15	6/10
BALB/cAnN	48±4	8/11
AKR/J	56±0	3/3
B10.A(2R)	56±0	1/1
C57BL/6N	65±2	9/13
DBA/1J	-	-
Control		
C3H/HeN	74±2	6/6
BALB/cAnN	74±2	6/6
AKR/J	80±9	6/7
B10.A(2R)	64±1	6/6
C57BL/6N	80±17	2/2
DBA/1J	42±3	0/8

[a]Mean ± standard error of the mean.
[b]IFA titer ⩾ 1:4.
Source: Walzer and Rutledge (1982).

mice, group B (steroid-treated), and Group C (steroid-tapered) mice and sacrificed weekly in a manner analogous to the protocol in rats. IgG was the principal antibody class found. Groups A and B mice sacrificed early in the study has no serum IgG antibodies to *P. carinii*. Serum antibody titers in group B rose slightly over time, but only reached a peak titer of 1:16 in one mouse. On the other hand, serum antibody titers increased noticeably in group C mice after steroids had been discontinued. Serum IgM antibodies were low or absent in all three groups of BALB/cAnN mice. The highest antibody titer found (1:16) occurred in a group B mouse at 4 weeks. IgA antibody titers were absent in almost all mice. The highest antibody titer noted was 1:4.

Table 13 summarizes the studies of serum antibodies to *P. carinii* among nude mice. The mice were exposed to various sources of *P. carinii* and their sera were tested to rat or mouse sources of the organism. Among the MSKCC Nu/Nu mice, serum antibodies of any immunoglobulin class were rare. IgG antibodies in low titer (1:4) were found in only three mice to rat *P. carinii,*

Table 13 Serum Antibodies to *P. carinii* in Nu/Nu and Nu/+ Mice

		Test source of *P. carinii*[a]					
			Rat			Mouse	
Group	Exposure	IgG[b]	IgM	IgA	IgG[b]	IgM	IgA
MSKCC							
Nu/Nu	Variable[c]	3/89	0/89	-	3/89	0/80	0/37
Kentucky							
Nu/Nu	Rat	0/82	0/82	0/77	0/82	0/82	0/63
Nu/+		19/40	5/40	0/32	4/40	0/40	0/23
Nu/Nu	Mouse	0/4	0/4	0/4	0/4	0/4	0/4
Nu/+		0/8	0/8	0/8	7/8	3/8	0/8
Nu/Nu	Control	0/23	0/23	0/22	0/23	0/23	0/22
Nu/+		0/16	0/16	0/16	0/16	1/16	0/15
BALB/cAnN							
Nu/+	Rat	1/12	0/12	0/12	8/12	2/12	0/12
Nu/+	Control	1/12	0/12	0/12	10/12	4/12	0/12

[a]No. positive (titer $\geq$ 1:4)/no. tested.
[b]Ig class of antibody.
[c]Includes exposure to rat and human *P. carinii* and controls.
Source: Walzer and Rutledge (1982).

and in 3 other mice to mouse *P. carinii.* These antibodies were unrelated to the type of exposure to the organism.

Kentucky Nu/Nu mice did not produce serum antibody of any immuno-globulin class, to rat or mouse *P. carinii.* On the other hand, 19 (48%) of 40 Nu/+ mice exposed to rat *P. carinii* produced serum IgG antibodies to the organism. All 19 mice had been injected with *P. carinii* infected rat lung homogenates. The peak serum IgG antibody titer was 1:32. Five of the mice produced serum IgM antibodies in low titer to rat *P. carinii,* and 4 also developed IgG antibodies in low titer to mouse *P. carinii.* Serum IgA anti-bodies were not detected.

The small number of Kentucky Nu/Nu mice exposed to mouse *P. carinii* did not produce serum antibody to rat or mouse sources of the organism. By contrast, 7 Nu/+ mice developed IgG antibodies and 3 Nu/+ mice developed IgM antibodies to mouse *P. carinii.* Control Kentucky Nu/Nu or Nu/+ mice rarely produced serum antibody to mouse or rat *P. carinii.*

As mentioned previously BALB/cAnN Nu/Nu and Nu/+ mice had been obtained in an attempt to establish a breeding colony and to study experimental *P. carinii* infection. Since the BALB/cAnN Nu/Nu males were in such poor health, only the Nu/+ females were used in the experimental infection studies and in studies of serum antibodies to *P. carinii*. As can be seen in Table 13 antibodies to rat *P. carinii* were rare in both control and exposed mice. However, antibodies to mouse *P. carinii* were very common among both groups of BALB/cAnN mice. These antibodies were primarily of the IgG class. The frequency of antibodies among these BALB/cAnN mice to mouse *P. carinii* may be due to the fact that subclinical *P. carinii* infection had been present among members of the mouse colony.

This study demonstrates that normal mice readily develop serum antibodies to mouse *P. carinii* detectable by the IFA technique. As with rats, the antibody levels in mice tended to be low with steroid administration and rose when steroids were discontinued; antibodies also developed in control mice through prolonged enviornmental exposure. IgG was the major immunoglobulin class found, as evidenced by both the frequency and level of the antibody titers. IgM antibodies were also present and in one mouse strain equaled or exceeded the IgG antibodies. IgA antibodies were uncommon and titers were low. In humans, IgG has been the major immunoglobulin class studied by the IFA technique (Brzosko et al., 1967; Lim et al., 1974; Meuwissen et al., 1977; Norman and Kagan, 1973; Pifer et al., 1978b; Shepherd et al., 1979); IgM antibodies have also been found but there has been little apparent interest in testing for IgA antibodies.

Serum antibody responses varied among the different strains of mice, but caution must be observed in interpreting thcse differences because of the small numbers of mice sometimes involved. Antibody responses did not appear to be related to the intensity of *P. carinii* infection. The lack of serum antibodies among DBA/1J mice also seemed to have less *P. carinii* infection. However, more detailed studies of this mouse strain need to be done before any firm conclusions can bc drawn.

Nu/Nu mice were unable to produce antibodies to *P. carinii*, whereas Nu/+ mice mounted a vigorous antibody response which was primarily of the IgG class. These data suggest that *P. carinii* antigens as measured by IFA require an intact functioning thymus for antibody production. Nu/Nu mice can respons to T-cell-independent antigens and produce IgM antibodies to a few organisms (Caulcy and Murphy, 1979; Iwasaki, 1978; Wortis, 1974), yet in most studies, IgG antibody responses have been lacking (Armstrong and Walzer, 1978). The fact that the outbred nude mice strains differed in their susceptibility to infection with *P. carinii* suggests that serum antibodies do not have a major role in host susceptibility or resistance to *P. carinii*. Studies of other inbred Nu/Nu mouse strains raised under similar environmental conditions would be helpful in clarifying the role of specific host immune factors to *P. carinii* infection. Finally, as in previous studies, the mice were able to distinguish between rat and mouse *P. carinii* in their antibody responses. This finding should be of help in studies of the basic biology of the *P. carinii* as well as in studies of host immune responses to the organism.

IX. Conclusion

Animal models have provided considerable insight about *P. carinii* infection but have significant limitations. At present there is no experimental animal which can be reliably infected with exogenous *Pneumocystis* organisms, whether derived from in vitro culture or from other animal sources. Such a system is necessary before standard techniques in infectious disease research can be applied to this organism. The following areas of *P. carinii* need to be defined: (1) dose-response curves (i.e., ranging from subclinical to lethal infection); (2) mode of infection (e.g., droplet nuclei, aspiration, etc.); (3) infective form of the organism (i.e., cyst or trophozoite); (4) incubation period. This system will then provide the basis for studies of pathogenesis of and host immune responses to the infection.

The relationship of *P. carinii* to host alveolar type 1 cells provides many opportunities for investigative work. In vitro methods such as tissue and organ culture might be developed to study the metabolism, attachment, and growth of *P. carinii* in a manner analogous to that of *M. pneumoniae* pneumonia.

3. Better methods must be developed for the quantitation of *P. carinii* and for isolation and purification of different stages (e.g., cyst, trophozoite) in the life cycle of the organism. There is a particular need to develop collaborative efforts between laboratories so that uniform and thus widely usable methods of identifying and quantitating organisms can be established. Efforts including in vitro cultivation and the production of specific antisera (e.g., monoclonal antibodies) would be helpful in this regard.

4. There is a pressing need to develop serologic tests for the detection of both *P. carinii* antigens and antibodies.

There is a need to study cellular immune function in *P. carinii* infection. This includes in vivo studies as well as in vitro models of lymphocyte-macrophage interaction.

Acknowledgment

This study was supported by the Medical Research Service, Veterans Administration, and a research grant from the American Cancer Society.

The author thanks Dr. Kokichi Yoneda for supplying electron microscopy photomicrographs.

References

Ammich, O. (1938). Uber die nichtsyphilitische interstitelle pneumonie des erstern kindesalters. *Virchows Arch. Pathol. Anat.* **302**:539-554.

Armstrong, D., and Walzer, P. (1978). Experimental infections in the nude mouse. In *The Nude Mouse in Experimental and Clinical Research.* (Edited by J. Fogh and B. C. Giovanella). New York, Academic Press, pp. 477-489.

Barnett, R. H., Hull, J. G., Vortel, V., and Schwarz, J. (1969). *Pneumocystis carinii* in lymph nodes and spleen. *Arch. Pathol.* **88**:175-180.

Barta, K. (1969). Complement fixation test for pneumocystosis. *Ann. Intern. Med.* **70**:235.

Bartlett, M. S., Vervanc, P. A., and Smith, J. W. (1979). Cultivation of *Pneumoxystis carinii* with WE-38 cells. *J. Clin. Microbiol.* **10**:796-799.

Barton, E. G., and Campbell, W. G. (1967). Further observations on the ultrastructure of pneumocystosis. *Arch. Pathol.* **83**:527-534.

Barton, E. G., and Campbell, W. G. (1969). *Pneumocystis carinii* in the lungs of rats treated with cortisone acetate. *Am. J. Pathol.* **54**:209-236.

Bazaz, G. R., Manfredi, O. L., Howard, R. G., and Claps, A. A. (1970). *Pneumocystis carinii* pneumonia in three full-term siblings. *J. Pediatr.* **76**:767-769.

Bazin, H., Beckers, A., and Querinjean, P. (1974). Three classes and four (sub) classes of rat immunoglobulins: IgM, IgA, IgE, and IgG_1, IgG_{2a}, IgG_{2b}, IgG_{2c}. *Eur. J. Immunol.* **4**:44.

Bowling, M. C., Smith, I. M., and Wescott, S. L. (1973). A rapid staining procedure for *Pneumocystis carinii. Am. J. Technol.* **39**:267-268.

Brody, A. R., Kelleher, P. C., and Craighead, J. F. (1978). A mechanism of exudation through intact alveolar epithelial cells in the lungs of cytomegalovirus infected mice. *Lab. Invest.* **39**:281-288.

Brzosko, W. J., Madalinski, K., and Nowoslawski, A. (1967). Fluorescent antibody and immunoelectrophoretic evaluation of the immune reaction in children with pneumonia induced by *Pneumocystis carinii. Exp. Med. Microbiol.* **19**:397-405.

Brzosko, W. J., Madalinski, K., Crawczynski, K., and Nowoslawski, A. (1971). Immunohistochemistry in studies on the pathogenesis of pneumocystis pneumonia in infants. *Ann. NY Acad. Sci.* **177**:156-170.

Burke, B. A., and Good, R. A. (1973). *Pneumocystis carinii* infection. *Medicine* **52**:23-51.

Campbell, W. G. (1972). Ultrastructure of *Pneumocystis* in human lungs: Life cycle of human pneumocystosis. *Arch. Pathol.* **93**:312-324.

Carini, A. (1910). Formas de eschizogonia do *Trypanozoma lewisi. Comm. Soc. Med. Sao Paolo* Aug. 16, p. 204.

Cauley, L., and Murphy, J. W. (1979). Response of congenitally athymic (nude) and phenotypically normal mice to *Cryptococcus neoformans* infections. *Infect. Immun.* **23**:644.

Chagas, C. (1909), Nova tripanozomiaza humana. *Mem. Inst. Oswaldo Cruz* **1**:159-218.

Chandler, F. W., Frenkel, J. K., and Campbell, W. G. (1979). Animal model: *Pneumocystis carinii* pneumonia in the immunosuppressed rat. *Am. J. Pathol.* **95**:571-574.

Chandler, F. W., McClure, H. M., and Campbell, W. G. (1967). Pulmonary pneumocystosis in nonhuman primates. *Arch. Pathol. Lab. Med.* **100**: 163-167.

Claman, H. N. (1972). Corticosteroids and lymphoid cells. *N. Engl. J. Med.* **287**:388-397.

Copland, J. W. (1974). Canine pneumonia caused by *Pneumocystis carinii*. *Aust. Vet. J.* **50**:515-518.

Csillag, A. (1957). Contributions to the taxonomical classification of the so-called *Pneumocystis carinii*. *Acta Microbiol. Acad. Sci. Hung.* **4**:1-8.

Decker, L. A. (Ed.). (1977). *Worthington Enzyme Manual*. Freehold, NJ, pp. 221-224.

DeJong, W. H., Steerenberg, P. A., Ursem, P. S., Osterhaus, A. D. M. E., Vos, J. G., and Ruitenberg, E. J. (1980). The athymic rat: III Natural cell-mediated cytotoxicity. *Clin. Immunol. Immunopathol.* **17**:163-172.

Delanoe, P., and Delanoe, M. (1912). Sur les rapporte des kystos de carinii le *Trypanosoma lewisi*. *Compt. Rend. Acad. Sci.* **155**:658-660.

Delanoe, P., and Delanoe, M. (1914). De la rarete de *Pneumocystis carinii* chez cobayes de la region de Paris; absense de kysts chez d'autres animaus lapin, grenouille, zanguilles. *Bull. Soc. Pathol. Exot.* **7**:271-274.

Dutz, W. (1970). *Pneumocystis carinii* pneumonia. *Pathol. Ann.* **5**:309-341.

Emmerling, P., Finger, H., and Bockemuhl, J. (1975). *Listeria* monocytogenes infection in mice. *Infect. Immun.* **12**:437-439.

Farrow, B. R. H., Watson, A. D. J., and Hartley, W. J. (1972). Pneumocystis pneumonia in the dog. *J. Comp. Pathol.* **82**:447-453.

Fough, J., and Giovenella, B. (Eds.). (1978). *The Nude Mouse in Experimental and Clinical Medicine*. New York, Academic Press.

Frenkel, J. K. (1976). *Pneumocystis jiroveci* n sp from man: Morphology, physiology, and immunology in relation to pathology. *Nat. Cancer Inst. Monogr.* **43**:13-30.

Frenkel, J. K., and Havenhill, M. A. (1963). The corticoid sensitivity of golden hamsters, rats, and mice. *Lab. Invest.* **12**:1402-1220.

Frenkel, J. K., Good, J. T., and Schultz, J. A. (1966). Latent pneumocystis infection of rats, relapse, and chemotherapy. *Lab. Invest.* 15:1559-1577.

Gabridge, M. G., and Taylor-Robinson, D. (1979). Interaction of *Mycoplasma pneumoniae* with human lung fibroblasts: Role of receptor sites. *Infect. Immun.* 25:455-459.

Gajdusek, D. C. (1957). *Pneumocystis carinii*–etiologic agent of interstitial plasma cell pneumonia of premature and young infants. *Pediatrics* 19: 543-565.

Gentry, L. O., Ruskin, J., and Remington, J. S. (1972). *Pneumocystis carinii* pneumonia. *Calif. Med.* 116:6-14.

Gleason, W. A., Roden, V. J., DeCastro, F. (1975). Pneumocystis pneumonia in Vietnamese infants. *J. Pediatr.* 87:1001-1002.

Goetz, O., and Rentsch, L. (1957). Weitere Untersuchungen zür experimentellen Rattenpneumocystose. *Z. Kinderheilk* 79:578-585.

Gold, J., L'Henreux, P., and Debner, L. P. (1977). Ultrastructure in the differential diagnosis of pulmonary histiocystosis and pneumocystosis. *Arch. Pathol. Lab. Med.* 101:243-247.

Gottschall, J. L., Walzer, P. D., and Yoneda, K. (1979). Morphological changes of the rat type II pneumocyte induced by oxytetracycline. *Lab. Invest.* 41:5

Ham, E. K., Greenberg, S. D., Reynolds, R. C., and Singer, D. B. (1971). Ultrastructure of *Pneumocystis carinii*. *Exp. Mol. Pathol.* 14:362-372.

Hashimoto, Y., Shigeru, T., Nisizawa, K., and Pigman, W. (1963). Action of proteolytic enzymes on purified bovine submaxillary mucin. *Ann. NY Acad. Sci.* 106:233-246.

Hellstrom, P. B., and Balish, E. (1979). Effect of tetracycline, the microbial flora, and the athymic state on gastrointestinal colonization and infection of BALB/c mice with *Candida albicans*. *Infect. Immun.* 23: 764-774.

Hendley, J. O., and Weller, T. H. (1971). Activation and transmission in rats of infection with *Pneumocystis carinii*. *Proc. Soc. Exp. Biol. Med.* 137:1401-1404.

Higuchi, H., Kameyama, K., and Kozima, K. (1972). One human case of *Pneumocystis carinii* infection and experimental pneumocystose in rats. *Jap. J. Thorac. Dis.* 10:515.

Hughes, W. T. (1979). Limited effect of trimethoprimsulfamethoxazole prophylaxis on *Pneumocystis carinii*. *Antimicrob. Agents Chemother.* 16:333-335.

Hughes, W. T., Kim, H. K., and Price, R. A. (1973). Attempts at prophylaxis for murine *Pneumocystis carinii* pneumonitis. *Curr. Ther. Res. Clin. Exp.* 15:581-587.

Hughes, W. T., Price, R. A., Sisko, F., Havron, W. S., Kafatos, A. G., Schonland, M., and Smythe, P. M. (1974a). Protein calorie malnutrition. *Am. J. Dis. Child.* **128**:44-52.

Hughes, W. T., McNabb, P. C., and Makres, T. D. (1974b). Efficacy of trimethoprim and sulfamethoxazole in the prevention and treatment of *Pneumocystis carinii* pneumonitis. *Antimicrob. Agents Chemother.* **5**: 289-293.

Hunninghake, G. W., Gudek, J. E., Kawanami, O., Ferrans, V. J., and Crystal, R. G., (1979). Inflammatory and immune processes in the human lung in health and disease: Evaluation by bronchiolalveolar lavage. *Am. J. Pathol.* **97**:149.

Hyun, B. H., Varga, C. F., Thalheimer, L. J. (1966). *Pneumocystis carinii* pneumonitis occurring in an adopted Korean infant. *JAMA* **195**:784-786.

Ikai, T. (1980). *Pneumocystis carinii:* Production of antibody either specific to trophozoite or to cyst wall. *Jpn. J. Parasitol.* **29**:115-126.

Ikai, T., Yoshida, Y., Ogino, K., Takeuchi, S., and Yamada, M. (1977). Studies on *Pneumocystis carinii* and *Pneumocystis carinii* pneumonia. II. Method for concentration and quantitation of *P. carinii* cysts. *Jpn. J. Parasitol.* **26**:314-322.

Iwasaki, Y. (1978). Experimental virus infections in nude mice. In *The Nude Mouse in Experimental and Clinical Research.* Edited by J. Fogh, and B. C. Giovanella. New York, Academic Press, p. 457.

Kelley, J., Landis, J. N., Davis, G., Trainer, T. D., Jakab, G. J., and Green, G. M. (1978). Diagnosis of pneumonia due to pneumocystis by segmental pulmonary lavage via the fiberoptic bronchoscope. *Chest* **74**: 24-28.

Kim, H. K., Hughes, W. T., and Feldman, S. (1972). Studies of morphology and immunofluorescence of *Pneumocystis carinii.* *Proc. Soc. Exp. Biol. Med.* **141**:304-309.

Kluge, R. M., Spaulding, D. M., and Spain, J. A. (1978). Combination of pentamidine and trimethoprimsulfamethoxazole in the therapy of *Pneumocystis carinii* pneumonia in rats. *Antimicrob. Agents Chemother.* **13**:975-978.

Kucera, K. (1967). Le pneumocystose en tant quanthropozoonose. *Ann. Parasitol.* **42**:565-581.

Lainson, R., and Shaw, J. J. (1975). Pneumocystis and histoplasma infections in wild animals from the amazon region of Brazil. *Trans. R. Soc. Trop. Med. Hyg.* **69**:505-508.

Lanken, P. N., Minda, M., Pietra, G. G., and Fishman, A. P. (1980). Alveolar response to experimental *Pneumocystis carinii* pneumonia in the rat. *Am. J. Pathol.* **99**:561-588.

Latorre, C. R., Sulzer, A. J., and Norman, L. G. (1977). Serial propagation of *Pneumocystis carinii* in cell line cultures. *Appl. Environ. Microbiol.* **33**:1204-1206.

Lim, S. K., Eveland, W. C., and Porter, R. J. (1973). Development and evaluation of a direct fluorescent antibody method for the diagnosis of *Pneumocystis carinii* infections in experimental animals. *Appl. Microbiol.* **26**:666-671.

Lim, S. K., Eveland, W. C., and Porter, R. J. (1974). Direct fluorescent-antibody method for the diagnosis of *Pneumocystis carinii* pneumonitis from sputa or tracheal aspirates from humans. *Appl. Microbiol.* **27**: 144-149.

Lim, S. K., Jones, R. H., and Eveland, W. C. (1971). Fluorescent antibody studies in experimental pneumocystosis. *Proc. Soc. Exp. Biol. Med.* **136**:675-679.

Linhartová, A. (1956). Experimentelle Pneumocystose bei Ratten. *Z. Bakt. I Abt. Orig.* **167**:178-186.

Linhartová, A. (1958). Weitere Beiträge zür experimentellen Lungen-pneumozystose. *Abl. Alleg. Pathol.* **98**:373-400.

Long, G. G., White, J. D., and Stookey, J. L. (1975). *Pneumocystis carinii* infection in splendectomized owl monkeys. *J. Am. Vet. Med. Assoc.* **167**:651-654.

Lozzio, B. B. (1976). The lasat mouse: A new model for transplantation of human tissues. *Biomedicine* **24**:144-147.

Masur, H., and Jones, T. C. (1978). The interaction in vitro of *Pneumocystis carinii* with macrophages and L-cells. *J. Exper. Med.* **147**:157-170.

McClure, H. M., Keeling, M. E., Custer, R. P., Marshak, R. R., Abt, D. A., and Ferrer, J. F. (1974). Erythroleukemia in two infant chimpanzees fed milk from cows naturally infected with bovine C-type virus. *Cancer Res.* **34**:2745-2757.

McConnell, E. E., Basson, P. A., and Pienaar, J. C. (1971). Pneumocystosis in a domestic goat. *Onderstepoort J. Vet. Res.* **38**.117-126.

McGhee, J. R., Michalek, S. M., and Ghanta, V. K. (1975). Rat immunoglobulins in serum and secretions: Purification of rat IgM, IgA, and IgG and their quantitation in serum, colostrum, milk and saliva. *Immunochemistry* **12**:817.

Meuwissen, J. H., and Leeuwenberg, A. D. (1972). A microcomplement fixation test applied to infection with *Pneumocystis carinii*. *Trop. Geogr. Med.* **24**:282-291.

Meuwissen, J., Leeuwenberg, A., and Heeren, J. (1973). New method for study of infections with *Pneumocystis carinii*. *J. Infect. Dis.* **127**:209-210.

Meuwissen, J. H. E., Tauber, I., Leeuwenberg, A. D. E. M., Beckers, P. J. A., and Sieben, M. (1977). Parasitologic and serologic observations of infection with *Pneumocystis* in humans. *J. Infect. Dis.* **136**:43–49.

Meyers, J. D., Pifer, L. L., Sale, G. E., and Thomas, E. D. (1979). The value of *Pneumocystis carinii* antibody and antigen detection for diagnosis of *Pneumocystis carinii* pneumonia after marrow transplantation. *Am. Rev. Respir. Dis.* **120**:1283-1287.

Milder, J. E., Walzer, P. D., Coonrod, J. D., and Rutledge, M. E. (1980). Comparison of histological and immunological techniques for the detection of *Pneumocystis carinii* in rat bronchial lavage fluid. *J. Clin. Microbiol.* **11**:409–417.

Minielly, J. A., McDuffie, F. C., and Holley, K. E. (1970). Immunofluorescent identification of *Pneumocystis carinii. Arch. Pathol.* **90**;561-566.

Minielly, J. A., Mills, S. D., and Holley, K. E. (1969). *Pneumocystis carinii* pneumonia. *Can. Med. Assoc. J.* **100**:846-854.

Mogensen, S. C., and Anderson, H. K. (1978). Role of activated macrophages in resistance of congenitally athymic nude mice to hepatitis induce by herpes simplex virus type 2. *Infect. Immun.* **19**:792-798.

Nakai, K., and Kamata, Y. (1974). Experimental studies of *Pneumocystis carinii* pneumonia. *The Saishin Igaku* **29**:399-407. (in Japanese).

Nickol, A. D., and Bonventure, P. F. (1977). Anomolous high native resistance of athymic mice to bacterial pathogens. *Infect. Immun.* **18**:636-645.

Nikolskii, S. N., and Shchetinin, A. N. (1967). *Pneumocystis* in swine. *Veterinariia* **44**:65.

Norman, L., and Kagan, I. G. (1973). Some observations on the serology of *Pneumocystis carinii* infections in the United States. *Infect. Immun.* **8**:317-321.

Norman, L., and Kagan, I. G., (1970). A preliminary report of an indirect fluorsecent antibody test for detecting antibodies to cysts of *Pneumocystis carinii* in human sera. *Am. J. Clin. Pathol.* **58**:170-176.

Ogino, K. (1978). *Pneumocystis carinii:* Experimental pulmonary infection in rats. *Jpn. J. Parasitol.* **27**:77-89.

Pavlica, F. (1962). The first observation of congenital pneumocystic pneumonia in a fully developed stillborn child. *Ann. Paediatr.* **198**:177-184.

Perera, D. R., Western, K. A., Johnson, H. D., Johnson, W. W., Schultz, M. G., and Akers, P. V. (1970). *Pneumocystis carinii* pneumonia in a hospital for children. *JAMA* **214**:1074-1078.

Pesanti, E. L. (1980). In vitro effects of antiprotozoan drugs and immune serum on *Pneumocystis carinii. J. Infect. Dis.* **141**:775-779.

Pifer, L., Hughes, W. T., and Murphy, M. J. (1977). Propagation of *Pneumocystis carinii* in vitro. *Pediatr. Res.* **11**:305-316.

Pifer, L. L., Hughes, W. T., Stagno, S., and Woods, D. (1978b). *Pneumo-*

cystis carinii infection: Evidence for high prevalence in normal and immunosuppressed children. *Pediatrics* **61**:35-41.

Pifer, L. L., Woods, D., and Hughes, W. T. (1978a). Propagation of *Pneumocystis carinii* in Vero cell culture. *Infect. Immun.* **20**:66-68.

Pliess, G., and Trode, H. (1958). Experimentelle Pneumocystose. *Frankf. Z. Pathol.* **69**:231-246.

Poelma, F. G. (1975). *Pneumocystis carinii* infections in zoo animals. *Z. Parasitenkd.* **46**:61-68.

Poelma, F. G., and Broekhuizen, S. (1972). *Pneumocystis carinii* in hares, *Lepus europaeus* Pallas, in the Netherlands. *Z. Parasitenkd.* **40**:195-202.

Price, R. A., and Hughes, W. T. (1974). Histopathology of *Pneumocystis carinii* infestation and infection in malignant disease in childhood. *Human Pathol.* **5**:737.

Reed, C., and O'Donoghue, J. L. (1982). The hairless athymic guinea pig. In *Proceedings of the Third International Workshop on Nude Mice.* Edited by N. D. Reed. New York, Gustav Fisher Verlag, pp. 51-57.

Ricken, J., and Remington, J. S. (1967). The compromised host and infection. I. *Pneumocystis carinii* pneumonia. *JAMA* **202**:1070-1074.

Rifkind, D., Faris, T. D., and Hill, R. D. (1966). *Pneumocystis carinii* pneumonia. *Ann. Intern. Med.* **65**:943-956.

Rosen, P., Armstrong, D., and Ramos, C. (1972). *Pneumocystis carinii* pneumonia. *Am. J. Med.* **53**:428-436.

Ruebush, T. K., Weinstein, R. A., Bachner, R. L., Wolff, D., Bartlett, M., Gonzales-Crussi, F., Silzer, A. J., and Schultz, M. G. (1978). An outbreak of pneumocystis pneumonia in children with acute leukemia. *Am. J. Dis. Child.* **132**:143-148.

Scher, I., Steinberg, A. D., Berning, A. K., and Paul, W. E. (1975). X-linked B-lymphocyte defect in CBA/n mice. *J. Exper. Med.* **142**:637-650.

Sheldon, W. H. (1959a). Subclinical pneumocystis pneumonitis. *Am. J. Dis. Child.* **97**:287-297.

Sheldon, W. H. (1959b). Experimental pulmonary *Pneumocystis carinii* infection in rabbits. *J. Exper. Med.* **100**:147-160.

Shepherd, V., Jameson, B., and Knowles, G. K. (1979). *Pneumocystis carinii* pneumonitis: A serological study. *J. Clin. Pathol.* **32**:773.

Shively, J. N., Dellers, R. W., Buergelt, C. D., Hsu, F. S., Kabelac, L. P., Moe, K. K., Tennant, B., and Vaughan, J. T. (1973). *Pneumocystis carinii* pneumonia in two foals. *J. Am. Vet. Med. Assoc.* **162**:648-652.

Shively, J. W., Moe, K. K., and Dellers, R. W. (1974). Fine structure of spontaneous *Pneumocystis carinii* pulmonary infection in foals. *Cornell Vet.* **64**:72-88.

Shultz, L., and Green, M. C. (1976). Motheaten, an immunodeficient mutant of the mouse. *J. Immunol.* **116**:936-1943.

Singer, C., Armstrong, D., Rosen, P. P., and Schottenfeld, D. (1975). *Pneumocystis carinii* pneumonia: A cluster of eleven cases. *Ann. Intern. Med.* **82**:772-777.

Solberg, C. O., Meuwissen, J. H., Needham, R. N., Good, R. A., and Matsen, J. M. (1971). Infectious complications in bone marrow transplant patients. *Br. Med. J.* **1**:18-23.

Stagno, S., Pifer, L. L., Hughes, W. T., Brasfield, D. M., and Tiller, R. E. (1980). *Pneumocystis carinii* in young immunocompetent infants. *Pediatrics* **66**:56-62.

Stahr, B. J., Walzer, P. D., and Yoneda, K. (1981). Effect of proteolytic enzymes on *Pneumocystis carinii* in rat lung tissue. *J. Parasitol.* **67**: 196-203.

Sueishi, D., Hisano, S., Sumiyoshi, A., and Tanaka, K. (1977). Scanning and transmission electron microscopic study of human pulmonary pneumocystosis. *Chest* **72**:213-216.

Tamura, T., Ueda, K., Furuta, T., Goto, Y., and Fujiwara, K. (1978). Electron microscopy of spontaneous pneumocystosis in a nude mouse. *Jpn. J. Exper. Med.* **48**:363-368.

Ueda, K., Goto, Y., Yamazaki, S., and Fujiwara, K. (1977). Chronic fatal pneumocystosis in nude mice. *Jpn. J. Exper. Med.* **47**:475-482.

Van de Meer, G., and Brug, S. L. (1942). Infection a Pneumocystis chez l'homme et chez les animaux. *Ann. Soc. Belg. Med. Trop.* **22**:301-307.

Vanden Akker, S., and Goldblood, E. (1960). Pneumonia caused by *Pneumocystis carinii* in a dog. *Trop. Geogr. Med.* **12**:54-58.

Vanek, J., and Jirovec, O. (1952). Parasitaere Pneumonie. Interstitielle plasmazellen Pneumonie der Fruehgeborenen verursacht durch *Pneumocystis carinii.* *Abl. Bakt.* **158**:120-127.

Vavra, J., and Kucera, K. (1970). *Pneumocystis carinii* Delanoe, its ultra-structure and ultrastructural affinities. *J. Protozool.* **17**:463-483.

Von Behren, L. A., and Pesanti, E. L. (1978). Uptake and degradation of *Pneumocystis carinii* by macrophages in vitro. *Am. Rev. Respir. Dis.* **118**:1051-1059.

Vos, J. G., Berkuens, J. M., and Kruijut, B. C. The athymic rat: I Morphology of lymphoid and endocrine organs. *Clin. Immunol. Immunopathol.* **15**:213-228.

Vossen, M. E. M. H., Beckers, P. J. A., Meuwissen, J. H. E., and Stadhoudeus, A. M. (1978). Developmental biology of *Pneumocystis carinii* and alternative view on the life cycle of the parasite. *A. Parasitenkd.* **55**:101-118.

Walzer, P. D. (1977). *Pneumocystis carinii* infection: A review. *South Med. J.* **70**:1130-1337.

Walzer, P. D., and Powell, R. D. (1982). Experimental *Pneumocystis carinii* infection in nude and steroid-treated normal mice. In *Proceedings of the Third International Workshop on Nude Mice.* Edited by N. D. Reed. New York, Gustav Fisher Verlag, pp. 123-132.

Walzer, P. D., and Rutledge, M. E. (1980). Comparison of rat, mouse, and human *Pneumocystis carinii* by immunofluorescence. *J. Infect. Dis.* **142**: 449.

Walzer, P. D., and Rutledge, M. E. (1981). Humoral immunity in experimental *Pneumocystis carinii* infection I: Serum and bronchial lavage fluid antibody responses in rats. *J. Lab. Clin. Med.* **97**:820-833.

Walzer, P. D., and Rutledge, M. E. (1982). Serum antibody responses to *Pneumocystis carinii* in different strains of normal and athymic (nude) mice. *Infect. Immun.* **35**:620-626.

Walzer, P. D., Powell, R. D., and Yoneda, K. (1979b). Experimental *Pneumocystis carinii* pneumonia in different strains of cortisonized mice. *Infect. Immun.* **24**:939-947.

Walzer, P. D., Yoneda, K., and Powell, R. D. (1980). Growth characteristics and pathogenesis of experimental *Pneumocystis carinii* pneumonia. *Infect. Immun.* **27**:928-937.

Walzer, P. D., Rutledge, M. E., Yoneda, K., and Stahr, B. J. (1979a). A new method of separating *Pneumocystis carinii* from infected lung tissue. *Exp. Parasitol.* **47**:356-368.

Walzer, P. D., Schnelle, V., Armstrong, D., and Rosen, P. P. (1977). Nude mouse: A new experimental model for *Pneumocystis carinii* infection. *Science* **197**:177-179.

Walzer, P. D., Schultz, M. G., Western, K. A., and Robbins, J. B. (1973). *Pneumocystis carinii* pneumonia and primary immune deficiency diseases of infancy and childhood. *J. Pediatr.* **82**:116-122. 122.

Walzer, P. D., Perl, D. P., Drogstad, D. J., Rawson, P. G., and Schultz, M. G. (1974). *Pneumocystis carinii* pneumonia in the United States. *Ann. Intern. Med.* **80**:83-93.

Wang, N. S., Huang, S. W., Thrulbeck, W. M. (1970). Combined *Pneumocystis carinii* and cytomegalovirus infection. *Arch. Pathol.* **90**:529-535.

Weber, W. R., Askin, F. B., and Dehner, L. P. (1977). Lung biopsy in *Pneumocystis carinii* pneumonia: A study of typical and atypical features. *Am. J. Clin. Pathol.* **67**:11-19.

Weller, R. W. (1956a). Zur Erzeugung von Pneumocystosen im Tierversuch. *Z. Kinderheilk* **76**:366-378.

Weller, R. W. (1956b). Weitere Untersuchungen über experimentelle Rattenpneumocystose im Hinblick auf die interstitelle Pneumonie der Frügebornen. *Z. Kinderheilk* **78**:166-176.

Western, K. A., Norman, N., and Kaufman, A. F. (1975). Failure of pentamidine isethionate to provide chemoprophylaxis against *Pneumocystis carinii* infection in rats. *J. Infect. Dis.* **131**:273-276.

Whitcomb, M. E., Schwarz, M. I., and Charles, M. A. (1970). Interstitial fibrosis after *Pneumocystis carinii* pneumonia. *Ann. Intern. Med.* **73**: 761-765.

Wortis, H. H. (1974). Immunological studies of nude mice. *Contemp. Topics Immunobiol.* **3**:243.

Yoneda, K., and Walzer, P. D. (1980). Interaction of *Pneumocystis carinii* with host lungs: An ultrastructural study. *Infect. and Immun.* **29**: 692-703.

Yoneda, K., and Walzer, P. D. (1981). Experimental *Pneumocystis carinii* pneumonia in the rat: Mechanism of alveolar injury. *Br. J. Exper. Pathol.* **62**:339-346.

Yoneda, K., and Walzer, P. D. (1983). Attachment of *Pneumocystis carinii* to type 1 alveolar cells: Study by freeze fracture electron microscopy. *Infect. Immun.* **40**:812-815.

Yoneda, K., Walzer, P. D., Richey, C. S., and Birk, M. G. (1982). *Pneumocystic carinii:* Freeze-fracture study of various stages of the organism. *Exper. Parasitol.* **53**:68-76.

Yoshida, Y., Ogino, K., Arizonon, N., Kodo, K., and Matsumo, K. (1974). Studies on *Pneumocystis carinii* and Pneumocystis pneumonia. (1) Appearance of this protozoa in cortisone treated rats. *Jap. J. Parasitol. (Suppl.)* **23** (in Japanese).

Yoshida, Y., Yanada, M., Shiota, T., Ikai, T., Takeuchi, S., and Ogino, K. (1981). *Pneumocystis carinii* in several kinds of animals. *Zbl. Bakt. Hyg.* **250**:206-212.

3

Interactions Between *Pneumocystis carinii* and Phagocytic Cells

HENRY MASUR

Clinical Center
National Institutes of Health
Bethesda, Maryland

I. Introduction

Pneumocystis carinii causes pneumonia almost exclusively in humans with abnormal immune function (Burke and Good, 1973; Walzer et al., 1974; Hughes, 1977). The vast majority of patients with pneumocystosis have multifaceted immunological dysfunction due to a combination of underlying disease process (often a malignant neoplasm), chemotherapy, and malnutrition, which makes it difficult to identify the relevant features of immune response against pneumocystis infection (Burke and Good, 1973; Walzer et al., 1974; Hughes, 1974; Hughes et al., 1974). A few patients with unusual isolated immune defects have permitted some insight into the components of immunity which are most important. Children with primary congenital immunodeficiency syndromes represent examples that pneumocystosis can be associated with isolated IgG or IgM deficiency, or with isolated T-lymphocyte dysfunction (Burke and Good, 1973; Walzer et al., 1973; DiGeorge, 1968). An unusual cluster of adult patients has shown that isolated T-lymphocyte dysfunction can also be associated with pneumocystosis; these are now recognized to have AIDS. Thus, cell-mediated and humoral immunity seem to have a key role in host defense against this infection. Pneumocystosis has not been associated with defects in quantity or quality of neutrophils or complement, by contrast, suggesting that these are not important factors with regard to anti-pneumocystis immune response.

The cellular response to pneumocystis infection that is seen histopathologically in the lung supports the concept that cell-mediated and humoral immunity are more important than neutrophil function. Essentially all humans, including those with normal neutrophil quantity and function, have a cellular pulmonary infiltrate that is exclusively mononuclear (Weber et al., 1977). In adults, lymphocytes are the predominant cell type, with moderate numbers of histiocytes, plasma cells, and alveolar macrophages (Weber et al., 1977). In the epidemic infantile form of the disease, plasma cells predominate. A neutrophil infiltration is not associated with pneumocystis pneumonia. A role for humoral response to *Pneumocystis* is supported by the plasma cell infiltration, and by the immunoglobulin coating which can be recognized on the intra-alveolar organisms (Brzosko et al., 1971).

Thus, the spectrum of susceptible patients and the histopathologic response suggest that cell-mediated and humoral immunity are important elements of host defense against pneumocystis infection. To understand the important mechanisms involved, an in vitro model has been established to assess individual components.

II. An In Vitro Model for Studying Pneumocystis-Mononuclear Phagocyte Interaction

Rats are a convenient animal for the investigation of *Pneumocystis* because they develop the disease spontaneously when treated with corticosteroids, and their lungs are large enough to manipulate. Furthermore, extensive literature exists concerning the response of *Pneumocystis* in rats after various immunologic or chemotherapeutic maneuvers (Frenkel et al., 1966; Chandler, et al., 1979). The model outlined below has previously been described in greater detail (Masur and Jones, 1978; Von Behren and Pesanti, 1978).

A. Methods and Materials

Collection of the Organisms and Cells

Sprague-Dawley rats spontaneously develop pneumocystis pneumonia 6-12 weeks after treatment with glucocorticosteroids. Effective regimens include adding 0.01 mg dexamethazone per milliliter of drinking water, or injecting the animals with 25 mg of cortisone acetate twice weekly. A low- (8%) protein diet enhances the severity of the illness. The addition of tetracycline,

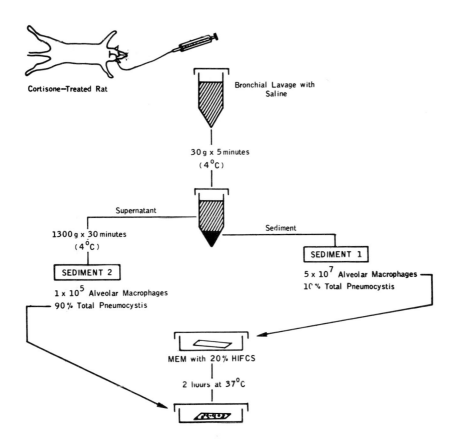

Figure 1 Technique for obtaining *Pneumocystis* and alveolar macrophages from a cortisone-treated rat. Eagle's minimum essential medium (MEM) and heat-inactivated fetal calf serum (HIFCS) were used to suspend the pellets.

1 mg and amphotericin B, 1 mg per milliliter of drinking water decreases the frequency of bacterial or fungal infection.

After the rat is sacrificed by intraperitoneal administration of pentobarbital (50 mg), the trachea is exposed aseptically and cannulated through a cervical incision with a 19-gauge polyethylene tube. The cannula is sutured into the trachea, and 50 cm^3 sterile saline is introduced in 5-10 cm^3 aliquots.

Figure 1 presents a schematic of the technique for separating the cellular components of bronchial lavage from the *Pneumocystis*. Differential centrifugation permits separation of a slow-speed sediment, which contains the majority of macrophages, and a high-speed sediment which contains most of the *Pneumocystis*.

Examination of the Bronchial Fluid

To determine if *Pneumocystis* are present, a drop of the high-speed sediment can be stained by Giemsa, toluidine blue O, Gram-Weigert, or methenamine silver techniques. The Giemsa technique is the only one which stains trophozoites as well as cysts. It is far more convenient, however, to examine the bronchial lavage fluid by phase contrast microscopy.

Culture of Mononuclear Phagocytic Cells

Rat alveolar macrophages are present in large numbers in the slow-speed sediment. The sediment from one animal is suspended in 4 cm^3 of Eagle's minimum essential medium (MEM) with 20% heat-inactivated fetal calf serum (HIFCS), and 0.5 ml of the suspension is then placed on 25 mm glass coverslips in 35 mm plastic tissue cultures dishes, and incubated for one hour at 37°C in 5% CO_2 to allow macrophages to adhere.

Mouse peritoneal macrophages, which are used in preference to rat peritoneal cells due to the large body of associated literature, are obtained by peritoneal lavage with 2-3 cm^3 of phosphate-buffered saline (PBS). The macrophages are then centrifuged at 30 g for 5 minutes, and resuspended in MEM-20% HIFCS. Then 1×10^6 cells are plated on 25 mm coverslips, incubated at 37°C in 5% CO_2 for 1 hour, and the nonadherent cells are removed by PBS washes. The adherent cells are then incubated overnight at 37°C in 5% CO_2.

Preparation of Anti-Pneumocystis Serum

Since *Pneumocystis* from one animal species may not be identical to *Pneumocystis* from other species, it is important to prepare the antiserum with organisms from the same animal species as those that are being used in the in vitro system (Frenkel et al., 1966; Walzer and Rutledge, 1980). For the rat model, sediment from the high-speed bronchial lavage centrifugation is assessed for pneumocystic content by phase contrast microscopy, and lyophilized. Rabbits are inoculated at three injection sites with 10 mg of lyophilized *Pneumocystis* suspended in distilled water and mixed with equal volumes of Freund's complete adjuvant. Fourteen days later, the same procedure is followed with Freund's incomplete adjuvant. The rabbit is bled 28 days after the initial inoculation, and the serum is heat inactivated, adsorbed with normal rat lung for 12 hours at 37°C, and stored at -20°C.

B. Identification of Macrophages and *Pneumocystis*

The lavage fluid of heavily infected animals contains as many as 10^9 pneumocystic organisms. The number depends on the severity of infection. Phase contrast microscopy reveals that the vast majority of organisms are round or oval, 3-6 μm in diameter, and have a thin phase-limiting membrane. Figure 2 shows these organisms, which are the trophozoite form, as they adhere to a rat alveolar macrophage under phase contrast microscopy. Many organisms also float freely in the suspension. The trophozoites can also be seen by light microscopy (Fig. 3), where they appear as dark blue-staining nuclei with small amounts of surrounding reddish cytoplasm.

Less than 1% of the *Pneumocystis* organisms in the bronchial lavage fluid are the cyst forms. The cyst form is 4-8 μ in diameter, has a thick, multilaminar, phase-dense-limiting membrane, and contains 4-8 phase-dense sporozoites. Figure 4 shows a cyst form in a phase contrast micrograph. In Figure 3, a light micrograph shows two cysts: with Giemsa stain, however, only the sporozoites can be visualized; the limiting membrane does not absorb the stain.

By phase contrast and light microscopy the sporozoite and the trophozoite appear morphologically similar. Electron micrographs show that the sporozoites are in fact much more electron-dense than are the trophozoites. Figure 5 shows an electron micrograph of a cyst form, with the electron-dense sporozoites. These electron-dense sporozoites are occasionally found in the bronchial lavage fluid, independent of the cyst wall. This suggests that the life cycle of *Pneumocystis* could include the sporozoites rupturing out of the cyst, and subsequently developing into trophozoites. Such a possibility is suggested by the electron micrograph in Figure 6, which could be interpreted as showing sporozoites rupturing out of the cyst, and becoming the less electron-dense trophozoites.

C. Interaction of Rodent Cells and *Pneumocystis*

When *Pneumocystis* organisms are added to monolayers of mouse fibroblasts, mouse peritoneal macrophages, or rat alveolar macrophages, they adhere readily to the surface of the rodent cells. They are not dislodged by vigorous washing. Figure 7 uses Nomarski micrography to demonstrate the extracellular location of the pneumocystic trophozoites with regard to mouse peritoneal macrophages. Figure 2 demonstrates the relationship of trophozoites to an alveolar macrophage by phase contrast microscopy. Addition of the trophozoites to freshly explanted rat alveolar macrophages, mouse peritoneal macrophages of any age, and L cells does not alter the morphology of the cells in terms of their spreading, their vacuoles and lipid bodies, or their ruffled membranes.

When trophozoites are added to freshly explanted rat alveolar macrophages, they are rarely ingested in the absence of anti-pneumocystis serum: they persist on the surface of the macrophage for several days. Prolonged

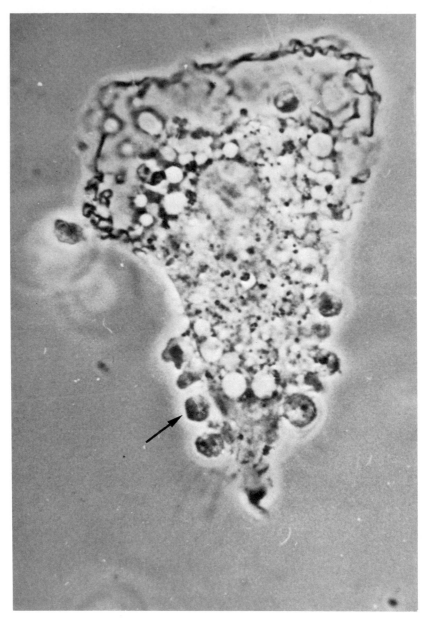

Figure 2 Phase contrast microscopic appearance of infected alveolar macrophages from a steroid-treated rat, cultured for 4 hours. The well-spread macrophage shows a central nucleus, lipid bodies, granules, multiple-phase lucent vacuoles, and a large ruffled edge of clear cytoplasm. Multiple pneumocystic trophozoites (arrow) are adherent to the surface of the macrophage (glutaraldehyde fixation, ×1200).

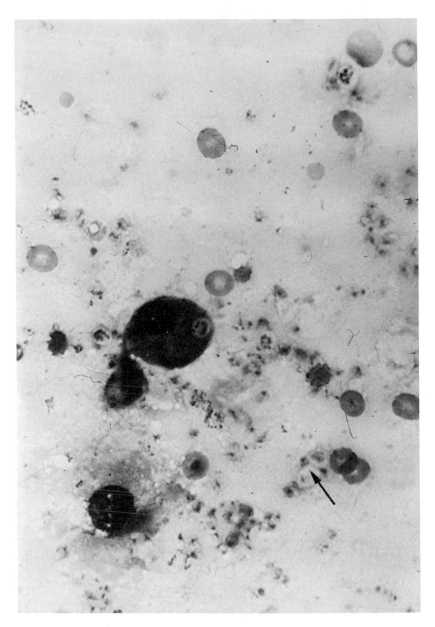

Figure 3 Light microscopic appearance of bronchial lavage sediment that is heavily infected with pneumocystic trophozoites. The trophozoites (arrow) are seen as seen as dark blue nuclei surrounded by a small amount of reddish cytoplasm. Two cyst forms can be identified (one in a macrophage vacuole): They appear as compact clusters of 4–8 sporozoites, each of which has an appearance similar to trophozoites by Giemsa stain (methanol fixation, ×630).

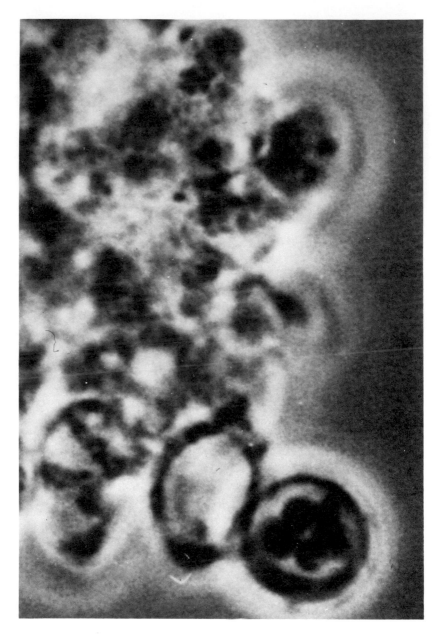

Figure 4 Phase contrast microscopic appearance of pneumocystic cyst, adjacent to a macrophage which is not in the plane of focus of this view. A total of 8 phase-dense sporozoites could be seen within the cyst wall by adjusting the planes of focus (glutaraldehyde fixation, ×1200).

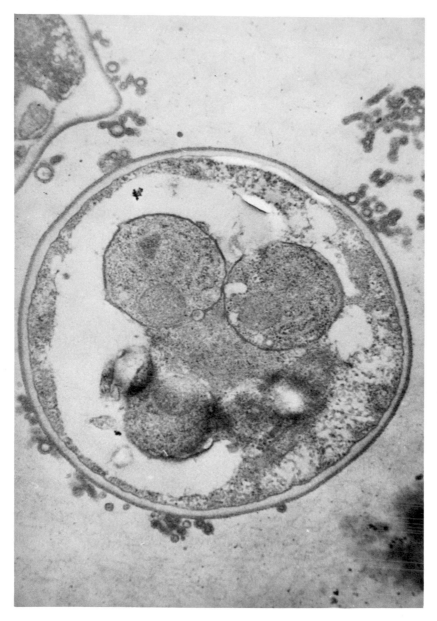

Figure 5 Electron microscopic appearance of pneumocystic cyst. The limiting membrane is composed of multiple layers. Tubular structures exterior to the limiting membrane can be seen in cross section. Other sections, not shown here, demonstrate that these arise from the cyst surface. The complex limiting membrane encloses electron-dense sporozoites, four of which can be seen here, each with its nucleus (×44,500).

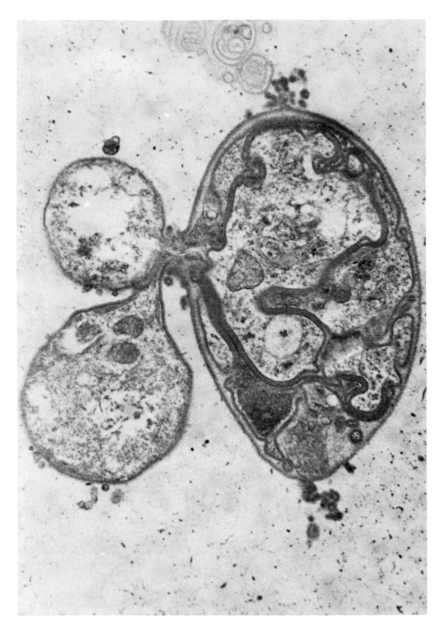

Figure 6   Electron microscopic appearance of pneumocystic cyst from which seem to be extruding forms that are more like trophozoites than the sporozoites seen in Figure 5. This suggests that the life cycle of *Pneumocystis* could include extrusion of the sporozoites from the cyst to become trophozoites (×44,500).

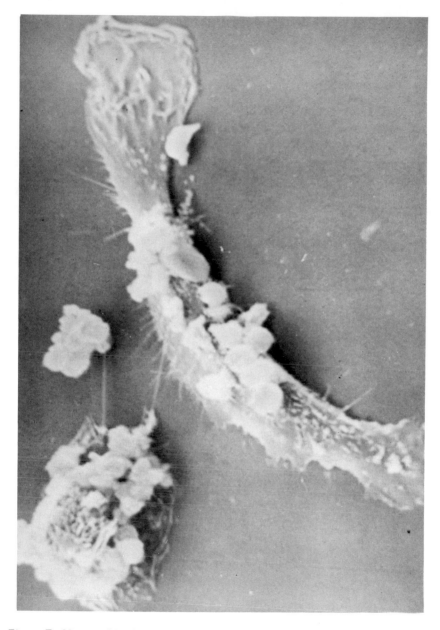

Figure 7 Normarski microgram demonstrates the extracellular location of pneumocystic trophozoites to two mouse peritoneal macrophages. The trophozoites are white, compact, oval or oblong bodies which can be seen covering sections of two macrophages, and also clumped in the glass coverslip between the two rodent cells ($\times$ 21,000).

observation of individual macrophages over many hours reveals an occasional trophozoite being interiorized into a vacuole, but over 95% remain on the surface membrane.

The addition of rabbit anti-pneumocystis serum to a heavily infected rat alveolar macrophage has a dramatic influence on the relationship of the organism to the rodent cell. Figure 8a shows a live heavily infected rat alveolar macrophage with many adherent trophozoites. Addition of normal rabbit serum induces no alteration in macrophage morphology or in trophozoite relationship to the macrophage surface. Figure 8b shows the same macrophage 30 minutes after the addition of rabbit anti-pneumocystis serum. Direct and continuous observation showed each trophozoite being interiorized and rapidly (within 2-4 min) degraded to an amorphous mass of phase-dense debris. Thus, in Figure 8b many empty vacuoles can be seen, but no organisms. The direct observation made it apparent that the effect of the anti-pneumocystis serum was not to detach or to destroy the trophozoites. The anti-pneumocystis serum had no effect on trophozoites which were adherent to the glass rather than to a cell, and no effect on uninfected macrophages, or on infected non-phagocytic cells (i.e., L cells). Figure 8c is an electron micrograph of a phagocytized trophozoite 15 min after addition of anti-pneumocystis serum.

These results suggest that *Pneumocystis* is an extracellular organism, much like mycoplasma, and that opsonization by freshly explanted rat alveolar macrophages requires specific antiserum. Once ingestion takes place, the organism is rapidly degraded, and there is no evidence for intracellular persistence or replication.

While the above observation has been confirmed, there have been some differences reported in the need for opsonic antiserum with mouse peritoneal macrophages and 48 hr in vitro cultivated rat alveolar macrophages. One

---

Figure 8 Phase contrast microscopic appearance of a living alveolar macrophage from a steroid-treated rat. The well-spread macrophage on the left (a) is shown 1 hr after infection with pneumocystic trophozoites. Numerous trophozoites (arrow) are shown adherent to the macrophage membrane. The same macrophage is shown on the right (b) 30 min after addition of anti-pneumocystis serum. Each trophozoite was directly observed to be interiorized by the macrophage into vacuoles. No adherent trophozoites remain and all engulfed trophozoites lost morphological characteristics within the vacuoles (X1500). (c) The electron microscopic appearance of a *Pneumocystis* organism (P) within a rat alveolar macrophage vacuole 15 min after the addition of anti-pneumocystis serum. Another vacuole (V) can also be seen surrounding electron-dense debris (X18,000).

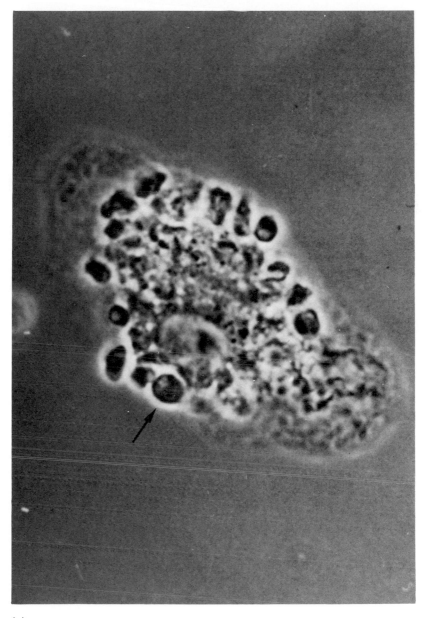

(a)

Figure 8

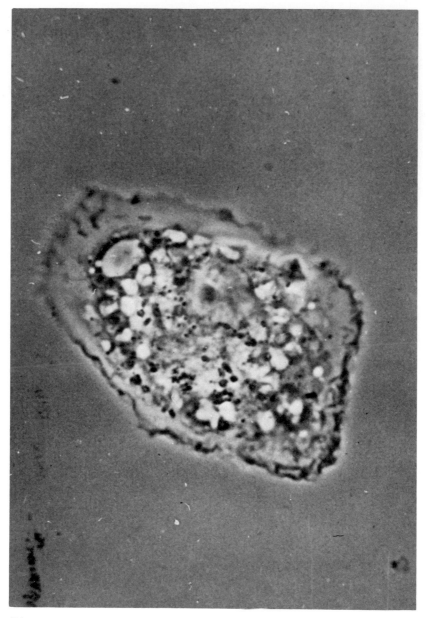

(b)

Figure 8   (continued)

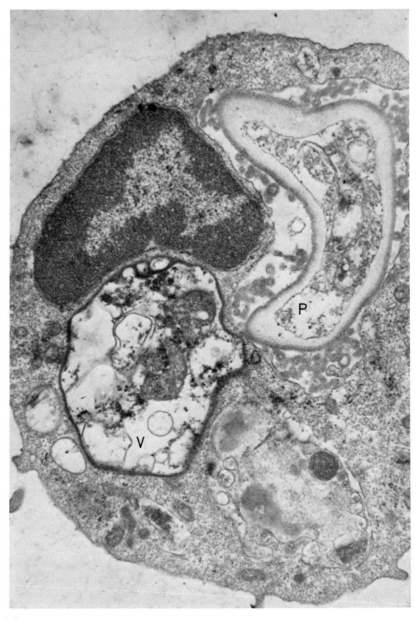

(c)

Figure 8   (continued)

laboratory has reported that mouse peritoneal macrophages of any age and two-day in vitro cultivated rat alveolar macrophages do not require antiserum for opsonization (Von Behren and Pesanti, 1978). Antiserum was required in work done at this laboratory (Masur and Jones, 1978). The differences may be due to technical considerations. The physiologic significance of any possible difference in phagocytic potential between freshly explanted and older cultivated alveolar macrophages is uncertain.

D. Effect of Pharmacologic Agents on *Pneumocystis* and on Rodent Cell-*Pneumocystis* Interaction

Some animals and some humans who develop pneumocystis pneumonia have circulating antibody and apparently intact mononuclear phagocytes (Lim et al., 1973; Norman and Kagan, 1973; unpublished data). Since many of these individuals are receiving chemotherapy at the time they develop pneumocystosis, an important question is how these chemotherapeutic agents predispose to pneumocystis pneumonia.

To determine if glucocorticosteroids interfere with the *Pneumocystis*-macrophage-antiserum system described above, alveolar macrophages from normal rats, glucocorticosteroid-treated rats without pneumocystosis, and glucocorticosteroid-treated rats with pneumocystosis were assessed. *Pneumocystis* trophozoites were added to each, and then rabbit anti-pneumocystis serum was added. These three macrophage populations showed no difference in the number of adherent trophozoites, the ability to interiorize the organism, or the ability to degrade the intravacuolar organisms. If hydrocortisone 100 μg/ml was added to the in vitro system using these three macrophage populations, no differences in these parameters could be detected. Thus, the effect of glucocorticosteroids to induce pneumocystis pneumonia does not appear to be affected through a disruption of antiserum opsonization, macrophage interiorization, or intravacuolar degradation. The effects of other chemotherapeutic agents have not been evaluated with this system.

The mechanisms by which chemotherapeutic agents alter the course of pneumocystis pneumonia are unknown. To assess whether these agents alter the relationship of *Pneumocystis* to mononuclear phagocytes, the effect of trimethoprim-sulfamethoxazole and pentamidine using this in vitro model have been examined (unpublished data). Concentrations of each drug comparable to pharmacologic serum concentrations were used: pentamidine 1-10 μg/ml; sulfamethoxazole 50-200 μg/ml. These drugs were added to heavily infected freshly explanted rat alveolar macrophages with rabbit anti-pneumocystis serum either present or absent. Observations over 24 hr revealed that these drugs had no effect on the morphology of *Pneumocystis* or macrophages, nor was the relationship between trophozoite and macrophage altered. Thus, these drugs did not cause lysis of the organism within 24 hr, nor could they replace anti-pneumocystis serum and induce phagocytosis of the organism. These results are consistent with in vivo data which suggest that neither trimethoprim-sulfamethoxazole nor pentamidine is microbicidal for *Pneumocystis* (Hughes, 1979; Western et al., 1975). These results also supplement studies on the effect of chemotherapeutic agents on supravital dye uptake by *Pneumocystis* (Pesanti, 1980). Neither pentamidine nor trimethoprim-sulfamethoxazole affects vital dye uptake rapidly: exposure of *Pneumocystis* for less than 6 hr has no effect. After 6 hr, pentamidine, but not trimethoprim-sulfamethoxazole, causes loss of *Pneumocystis'* ability to concentrate the dye. More informative studies on the mechanism of action of these drugs on *Pneumocystis* will require a system for in vitro cultivation of the organism.

III. Interactions Between *Pneumocystis* and Human Phagocytic Cells

Very little work has been done to assess the interaction of *Pneumocystis* with human mononuclear phagocytes and neutrophils. Preliminary work has shown that *Pneumocystis* readily adhere to both types of human cells. More information is needed, however, about the reliability with which these cells interiorize and degrade *Pneumocystis*. A comparison of the anti-pneumocystis activity of these circulating cells would be particularly interesting in comparison with the anti-pneumocystis activity of human alveolar macrophages since *Pneumocystis* is a disease which (with rare exceptions) is confined exclusively to the lungs. Such data are not yet abailable.

IV. Summary and Conclusion

In vitro studies have demonstrated that *Pneumocystis* organisms are abundant in bronchial lavage fluid. The trophozoite is the most frequent pneumocystis form observed; cysts are relatively uncommon. The trophozoites adhere readily to phagocytic cells and fibroblasts. Rabbit anti-pneumocystis serum is required for freshly explanted rat alveolar macrophages to ingest *Pneumocystis*. Nonimmune serum, complement, pentamidine, trimethoprim-sulfamethoxazole, and glucocorticosteroids have no effect on the morphology of the trophozoites, or their relationship to phagocytic cells. Once the *Pneumocystis* are interiorized, they are rapidly degraded, suggesting that in this model there is no intracellular stage in the life cycle of *Pneumocystis*.

These studies would suggest that intact antibody response and mononuclear phagocyte function are required for adequate host defense against *Pneumocystis*. Thus, patients with inadequate antibody synthesis, or inadequate phagocyte function may develop pneumocystosis (Burke and Good, 1973; Walzer et al., 1974; Hughes, 1977; Pedersen et al., 1979). Since animals and humans who have fulminant pneumocystis pneumonia often have apparently intact mononuclear phagocyte function and circulating anti-pneumocystis antibody, as well as an abundant pulmonary infiltrate with mononuclear cells and antibody-coated *Pneumocystis,* other factors must be involved. Further studies of cell-mediated immune phenomena are necessary, with particular attention directed at factors unique to the lungs, since this infection rarely involves extrapulmonary sites. These studies will be greatly facilitated if *Pneumocystis* can be adequately cultured in vitro so that a source of pure antigen is available, and the effects of various manipulations on the proliferating organism can be studied.

References

Brzosko, W. J., Madalinski, K., Krawczynski, K., and Nowoslawski, A. (1971). Immunohistochemistry in studies on the pathogenesis of pneumocystis pneumonia in infants. *Ann. N.Y. Acad. Sci.* **177**:156-170.

Burke, B. A., and Good, R. A. (1973). *Pneumocystis carinii* infection. *Medicine* **52**:23-51.

Chandler, F. W., Frenkel, J. K., and Campbell, W. G. (1979). Animal model: *Pneumocystis carinii* pneumonia in the immunosuppressed rat. *Am. J. Pathol.* **95**:571-574.

DiGeorge, A. M. (1968). Congenital absence of the thymus and its immunological consequences: Occurrence with congenital hypoparathyroidism. In *Immunologic Deficiency Diseases in Man.* Birth Defects Original Article Series. Edited by R. A. Good and D. Bergsma. National Foundation Press.

Frenkel, J. K., Good, J. T., and Schultz, J. A. (1966). Latent *Pneumocystis* of rats, relapse, and chemotherapy. *Lab. Invest.* **15**:1559-1577.

Hughes, W. T. (1977). Pneumocystis pneumonia. *N. Engl. J. Med.* **297**: 1381-1383.

Hughes, W. T. (1979). Limited effect of trimethoprim-sulfamethoxazole prophylaxis on *Pneumocystis carinii. Antimicrob. Agents Chemo.* **16**: 333-335.

Hughes, W. T., Price, R. A., Sisko, F., Havron, W. S., Kafatos, A. G., Schonland, M., and Smythe, P. M. (1974). Protein-calorie malnutrition—a host determinant for *Pneumocystis carinii* infection. *Am. J. Dis. Child.* **128**:44-52.

Lim, S. K., Eveland, W. C., and Porter, R. J. (1973). Development and evaluation of a direct fluorescent-antibody method for the diagnosis of

Pneumocystis carinii infections in experimental animals. *Appl. Microbiol.* **26**:666-671.

Masur, H., and Jones, T. C. (1978). The interaction in vitro of *Pneumocystis carinii* with macrophages and L-cells. *J. Exp. Med.* **147**:157-170.

Norman, L., and Kagan, I. G. (1973). Some observations on the serology of *Pneumocystis carinii* infections in the United States. *Infect. Immun.* **8**:317-321.

Pedersen, F. K., Johansen, K. S., Rosenkvist, J., Tygstrup, I., and Valerius, N. H. (1979). Refractory *Pneumocystis carinii* infection in chronic granulomatous disease: Successful treatment with granulocytes. *Pediatrics* **64**:935-938.

Pesanti, E. L. (1980). In vitro effects of antiprotozoan drugs and immune serum on *Pneumocystis carinii. J. Infect. Dis.* **6**:775-780.

Von Behren, L. A., and Pesanti, E. L. (1978). Uptake and degradation of *Pneumocystis carinii* cy macrophages in vitro. *Am. Rev. Respir. Dis.* **118**:1051-1059.

Walzer, P. D., and Rutledge, M. E. (1980). Comparison of rat, mouse, and human *Pneumocystis carinii* by immunofluorescence. *J. Infect. Dis.* **142**:449.

Walzer, P. D., Schultz, M. G., Western, K. A., and Robbins, J. B. (1973). *Pneumocystis carinii* pneumonia and primary immune deficiency diseases of infancy and childhood. *J. Pediatr.* **82**:416-422.

Walzer, P. D., Perl, D. P., Krogstad, D. J., Rawson, P. G., and Schultz, M. G. (1974). *Pneumocystis carinii* pneumonia in the United States. *Ann. Intern. Med.* **80**:83-93.

Weber, W. R., Askin, F. B., and Dehner, L. P. (1977). Lung biopsy in *Pneumocystis carinii* pneumonia—a histopathologic study of typical and atypical features. *Am. J. Clin. Pathol.* **67**:11-19.

Western, K. A., Norman, L., and Kaufman, A. F. (1975). Failure of pentamidine isethionate to provide chemoprophylaxis against *Pneumocystis carinii* infection in rats. *J. Infect. Dis.* **131**:273-276.

4

Serology of *Pneumocystis carinii*

BERYL JAMESON

Royal Marsden Hospitals
London, England

I. Introduction

Serological investigations of *Pneumocystis carinii* pneumonitis are still in their infancy. In general, studies indicate that *P. carinii* infections occur frequently as mild or subclinical acquisitions, probably early in life, and that the appearance of the severe infection which has in recent years been associated with an immunocompromised host is reactivated latent disease.

Early work in Europe employed complement fixation methods when studying the epidemic form of disease which occurred in conditions of overcrowding and malnutrition. Subsequent investigations suggest that these methods may not be appropriate to the hypoimmune patient.

This chapter is a sequential account of published methods and results, with their conclusions from the past twenty years, but mostly from the past decade. A synopsis appears in Table 1. None can yet be said to show close agreement and this is unfortunately compounded by the fact that the excellent success rate of treatment with high-dose trimethoprim-sulfamethoxazole (Hughes et al., 1975; Lau and Young, 1976) has led to a decline in histological confirmation of the infection. That is, a test of response to treatment has in many instances been substituted for diagnostic procedures such

Table 1 Synopsis of Antibody Studies Quoted

Reference	Method	Antigen	Subjects	Principle conclusions
Barta, 1969	CFT[a]	-	119 Cases (Epidemic type); 120 controls	CFT valuable in immunocompetent subjects
Nowoslawski and Brzosko, 1964	IF[b]	Tissue section	6 Infected infants (epidemic type)	IF as good as CFT
Brzosko et al., 1967	IF	Tissue section	37 Cases (epidemic type)	IgM and IgG antibody formed
Brzosko et al., 1971	IF	Tissue section	4 Infected infants aged 11–15 weeks	Exudate in lungs consists of IgG and IgM
Norman and Kagan, 1972, 1973	IF	Cyst suspensions, rat and human origin	191 Cases (hypoimmune); 109 contacts; 74 noncontacts	44% cases positive at 1:8 titer 1:20 indicative of active infection
			Serial sera from 53 cases	No diagnostic pattern of antibody response
				No difference in either antigen
Meuwissen et al., 1977	IF	Cyst suspensions, human origin	600 Normal; 117 children with acute lymphoblastic leukemia	Nearly 100% of children are infected during the first 2 years of life

Pifer et al., 1978	IF	Cysts grown in vitro on chicken embryo lung	Serial sera from children (birth to 7 years)	63% of Children have been infected by the age of 4
Pintozzi, 1978	IF	Cysts from rats	Hypoimmune patients	Immunoglobulins IgG and IgA (compare epidemic form); Absence of IgM explains failure of CFT
Shepherd et al., 1979	IF	Tissue section	91 Controls, 23 patients (hypoimmune)	56% controls positive IgG up to 1:32 of cases: 10 above 1:32 5 fourfold rise within 1:32 Useful diagnostic value
Ikai, 1980	IF	Trophozoite (T) and cyst	Tissue sections (containing both elements) and cysts	T antibody positive on tissue section but not on cyst suspension Possible explanation of varying results when different substrates used

[a]Complement fixation test.
[b]Indirect immunofluorescence.

as lung biopsy. Consequently, it is difficult to exclude false-positive serology because the therapeutic spectrum of trimethoprim-sulfamethoxazole extends well beyond pneumocystis infection. Reasons for variable findings include differences in technique and interpretation, the immune status of the studied groups and, above all lack of antigen in the form of pneumocysts cultured in vitro. What follows, therefore, is a chronological account of the emergence of serological methods.

II. History of Available Literature

Barta (1969) reviewed the results of complement fixation tests on more than 1300 sera collected between 1952 and 1965. Complement-fixing antibodies were found in 90% of 119 histologically proven fatal cases, compared with only 3% of a control group of 120 cases of pneumonitis due to other causes. Seropositivity was also found in 75-85% of young children with clinically suspected disease. These children were immunocompetent. The apparent superiority of immunofluorescence (IF) in the hypoimmune patient is presumably due to absence of increased complement-fixing IgM.

Nowoslawski and Brzosko (1964) used IF in a study of an outbreak of the infection in Warsaw during May and June of 1963. The indirect procedure was used on formalin-fixed sections of infected lung. This was later refined by using a fixative which destroyed the human globulin in alveolar exudate, while preserving the polysaccharide antigen of the pneumocyst, thereby improving the stain specificity. The authors presented the conclusion that this method was at least as reliable as complement fixation. Six serological samples from infected infants were tested and all produced a brilliant fluorescence in the alveolar spaces which were, characteristically, stuffed with cysts. This was quite distinguishable from any autofluorescence from the rest of the tissue. It is of interest that a "substantial decrease" of fluorescence occurred after 1:32 dilution of all the sera.

They also examined sera from 37 infants below the age of two years with no apparent respiratory disease. In contrast to later publications, only two sera from this group gave a positive result for pneumocystis antibody. Three of 13 infants with mild respiratory symptoms who were in the hospital at the time of the outbreak were seropositive, and in their discussion the authors comment on the presence in the population of asymptomatic carriers of infection.

Work from the same source (Brzosko et al., 1967) investigated the incidence of IgM and IgG antibody in 37 children of whom 17 had died from the infection, 16 had clinical and radiological evidence of pneumocystosis, and 4 had a history of the infection some months previously. IgM antibodies alone were found in six children who were less than eight weeks old. Combinations of IgM and IgG were found in 18 who were between three and six months of age. In the remaining 13, who were all over two months old, only IgG antibody was found.

Yet more Polish studies (Brzosko et al., 1971) comprised a comprehensive study of necropsy material from four infants aged 11-15 weeks. All were full-term births and had no congenital abnormality or hypogammaglobulinemia. As the result of application of immunohistochemical techniques they demonstrated that the typical foamy exudate in the alveolar spaces consisted of pneumocysts found with IgG and IgM, but only trace amounts of IgA. It was inferred that children who died from the "epidemic infantile" form of the disease had no impairment of immunoglobulin synthesis, but that there was a significant delay in binding of complement by immune complexes which was related to the young age of the susceptible subjects.

Norman and Kagan (1972, 1973) directed their attention to the "hypoimmune, hypoergic" type of patient, in whom the infection occurs in sporadic rather than epidemic form and is the result of natural or drug-induced impaired immunity. Also, instead of using fixed tissue sections, the antigen for their immunofluorescent (IF) stains consisted of pneumocysts from either rat or human lung, prepared in suspension by a process of homogenization, filtration, and passage through a discontinuous sucrose gradient. The suspensions were air dried on microscope slides and stored at -70°C. Immunofluorescence procedures were compared with complement fixation tests.

Sera were tested by IF from 58 confirmed cases, 133 clinically suspected cases, 109 healthy contacts, and 74 healthy noncontacts. At a titer of 1:8, the percentage of seropositives was the same in the confirmed and suspected cases: that is 26/58 (44.8%) of the former and 59/133 (44.4%) of the latter. Of the 109 healthy contacts, eight (7.3%) were positive and only one (1.4%) of the noncontacts. At a titer of 1:20 the noncontacts were all negative and it was suggested that this titer was indicative of active infection, although this arbitrary conclusion was not supported by a further study on 437 people without pneumocystis pneumonitis, but with other illnesses, mostly malignancies. At a 1:8 dilution 267/437 (61.1%) were found positive and 82 of these (18.7%) were still seropositive at 1:20. Furthermore, having tested 120 serial specimens from 53 proven cases they concluded that they could not demonstrate a pattern of antibody appearance, during or after infection, which was of either immediate or retrospective diagnostic value. This is at variance with the reports of later workers and the authors also comment that the rate of serological positivity is disappointingly low compared with that reported during European epidemics. As mentioned at the beginning of the chapter, these conflicting findings can perhaps be related to the different immune status of the patients under investigation, but it seems also that, as will be shown later, varying techniques contribute to the lack of reproducibility of results.

They found no difference in the usefulness of antigen prepared by their method from either human or rat lung, although using tissue sections, steroid-induced rat infections appear to be less useful owing to the more diffuse distribution of infection in the rat lung, which makes it more difficult to obtain a clear end point (unpublished). Their finding that, in contrast to studies on marasmic infants in epidemics, the antibody found in healthy persons and patients with sporadic infection was of the IgG class supports the opinion that latent infection might become reactivated by immunosuppression.

In the Netherlands (Meuwissen et al., 1977), pronase-treated cyst suspensions from human lung were used in an IF investigation from which it was concluded that nearly 100% of children are infected by *P. carinii* during the first two years of life. In the United States (Pifer et al., 1978), it was reported that about 75% of children have acquired the infection by the age of four. In this instance the antigen used for the IF method was *P. carinii* organisms propagated in vitro on chick embryo lung (Pifer et al., 1977). Groups of individuals studied included normal children and cancer patients with and without proven pneumocystis pneumonitis.

At the same time, these workers tested for antigenemia using counter-immunoelectrophoresis (CIE). Antibody used in the test was produced in rabbits by injection of pneumocysts derived from either human or murine sources, or in soluble form (Meyers et al., 1979). The sera were absorbed with a variety of agents which included infected and normal lung, *Candida albicans, Escherichia coli* and *Staphyloccoccus aureus,* to test for specificity. No precipitin bands were found with sera from 120 normal children nor from eight leukemic children who were receiving prophylactic trimethoprim-sulfamethoxazole, which has been found to be a highly effective preventive measure. On the other hand, positive reactions occurred in 19 of 20 *fresh* sera from proven cases and in 64 of 103 (62%) sera from proven cases which had been stored at -70°C for up to five years.

Although such findings have yet to be reproduced by other workers, the possibility of detecting antigenemia offers much potential for diagnosis, since no one would willingly subject a patient suffering extreme respiratory distress to invasive histological investigation if an alternative were available.

This same group of workers were especially fortunate in having access to serial sera which had been collected in a group of children from birth up to the age of seven years. Seropositivity (apart from that which might reflect maternal transfer) began at seven months old and was present in 63% by the age of four. The variance in age distribution from that suggested by Meuwissen and his co-workers (1977) could be accounted for by such factors as the highly subjective nature of IF techniques and the fact that the American sera had been in long-term store. However, there could also be geographical differences, such as are seen in reverse in the prevalence of fungal opportunistic infections when Europe and North America are compared.

Pintozzi (1978), using cysts obtained from rats in which the infection was induced by immunosuppression with corticosteroids, reported that the host immunoglobulins on the cyst surface were predominantly IgG and IgA. Since this differs from the findings of Brzosko et al. (1967, 1971) mentioned earlier in the chapter, he concludes that this may explain why complement fixation methods appear to have been more successful in the infantile epidemic form of disease than in the hypoimmune type. Large amounts of IgM found in the former would aid complement fixation.

Bone marrow transplantation, which may involve a severely immunosuppressive condition, for example with both cytotoxic drugs and whole body irradiation, has been frequently complicated by late-onset pneumonitis (at days 30-100). The most common infecting agents are *Pneumocystis* and cytomegalovirus, though many cases are idiopathic. A group of bone marrow recipients have been tested for the presence of pneumocystis antigen, using the method described above (Meyers et al., 1979). Although antigen was only demonstrated in 1/50 marrow donors, antigenemia among recipients was reported in 79% of 28 cases of proven pneumocystosis, 69% of 26 cases of viral pneumonitis, and 79% of 28 patients with undiagnosed pulmonary infiltrates.

Although this is disappointing in terms of failing to provide a reliable noninvasive diagnostic method, it could be held to support the view that subclinical infection is more common than has been appreciated until recently. If this technology can be reproduced by other workers it may be hoped that perhaps a quantitative element might usefully be introduced.

III. Serological Studies in the United Kingdom

The first serological study published in the United Kingdom (Shepherd et al., 1979) resulted from an apparent outbreak of *P. carinii* pneumonitis in an oncology unit. Starting in November 1974, 32 cases occurred over a period of 34 months. By contrast in the same hospital, only three cases had been detected in the previous ten years. In fact, at that time, *P. carinii* infections were still regarded as a rarity nationwide. The 32 cases comprised 13 which were histologically proven and 19 who were diagnosed on the grounds of clinical presentation, chest radiograph appearance, and response to specific therapy: pentamidine isethionate or later, high-dose trimethoprim-sulfamethoxazole. Their ages ranged from 4-52 years and acute lymphoblastic leukemia predominated (15 patients).

Serology was performed on 23 of the 32 patients, using IF with tissue sections of heavily infected lung as the substrate. In fact, the tissue came from the same source as that used by Nowoslawski and Brzosko (1964), generously donated by the National Institute of Hygiene in Warsaw. Admission and serial convalescent sera (up to eight samples) were tested. The results were compared with single sera obtained from 31 family contacts and 60 healthy noncontacts.

The two groups of nonpatients gave the same results: 56% positive, the highest titer being 1 in 32. In the group of patients, 10 achieved maximum titers above the "normal" limit of 1 in 32 (up to 1 in 128); five showed a fourfold rise within the "normal" limit; three converted from negative to positive at 1 in 8; one proven case remained negative. Two died when only admission specimens had been collected. Two clinically suspected cases did not show rising titers. They were treated with high-dose trimethoprim-sulfamethoxazole which may have been effective against micro-organisms other than *P. carinii.*

Therefore, 18 of the 21 evaluable cases were regarded as having seroconverted. In all instances the antibody was of the IgG class with no rise of IgM. Maximum levels were demonstrable at 10-14 days after admission to hospital.

In addition to adding support to previous observations which suggest reactivated latent infection in immunosuppressed patients, the authors of this paper conclude that serology has a useful role in the diagnosis and management of infections. Some of the patients studied had antibody titers above the accepted normal range at the time of hospital admission and the presence of high or rising antibody levels may assist the decision to continue treatment in the face of side effects.

Since the publication of this small series of cases, over 500 sera have been examined from various hospitals in the United Kingdom. Full clinical details are not always available, but (unpublished) observations continue to sustain this opinion. In particular there is strong evidence that false positive results do not occur, although negative results have been obtained in some heavily immunosuppressed patients. Specificity of testing is indicated by the fact that brilliant fluorescence is confined to the alveolar spaces where the pneumocysts are most abundant. (other micro-organisms would be more likely to be found in the lung tissue.) Nevertheless, there is a need for a source of pure antigen obtained from in vitro culture of pneumocysts to confirm these findings.

IV. Conclusions

The growing interest in pneumocystic serology as yet has not produced much uniformity of assessment. This must in some part be due to the wide variety of techniques used for preparing antigen. Ikai (1980) has compared cyst-derived with trophozoite-derived antigen and shown them to differ. This could explain some of the differences between methods using tissue sections, which contain both forms, and purified cyst suspensions.

There is clearly a long way to go before serological methods find a definitive place in the study of the natural history of this increasingly important disease.

References

Barta, K. (1969). Letter. *Ann. Int. Med.* **70**:235.

Brzosko, W., Madalinski, K., and Nowoslawski, A. (1967). Fluorescent antibody and immunoelectrophoretic evaluation of the immune reaction in children with pneumonia induced by *Pneumocystis carinii. Exp. Med. Microbiol.* **19**:397-405.

Brzosko, W. J., Madalinski, K., Krawczynski, K., and Nowoslawski, A. (1971). Immunohistochemistry in studies on the pathogenesis of pneumocystis pneumonia in infants. *Ann. N.Y. Acad. Sci.* **117**:156-170.

Hughes, W. T., Feldman, S., and Sanyal, S. K. (1975). Treatment of *Pneumocystis carinii* pneumonitis with trimethoprim-sulphamethoxazole. *Canad. Med. Assoc. J.* **112**:475-505.

Ikai, T. (1980). *Pneumocystis carinii:* Production of antibody either specific to trophozoite or cyst wall. *Jpn. J. Parasitol.* **29**:115-126.

Lau, W. K., and Young, L. S. (1976). Trimethoprim-sulfamethoxazole treatment of *Pneumocystis carinii* pneumonia in adults. *N. Engl. J. Med.* **295**:716-718.

Meuwissen, J. H. E. Th., Tauber, I., Leeuwenberg, A. D. E. M., Beckers, P. J. A., and Sieben, M. (1977). Parasitologic and serologic observations of infection with *Pneumocystis* in humans. *J. Infect. Dis.* **136**:43-49.

Meyers, J. D., Pifer, L. L., Sale, G. E., and Thomas, E. D. (1979). The value of *Pneumocystis carinii* antibody and antigen detection for diagnosis of *Pneumocystis carinii* pneumonia after marrow transplantation. *Am. Rev. Respir. Dis.* **120**:1283-1287.

Norman, L., and Kagan, I. A. (1972). A preliminary report of an indirect fluorescent antibody test for detecting antibodies to cysts of *Pneumocystis carinii* in human sera. *Am. J. Clin. Pathol.* **58**:170-176.

Norman, L., and Kagan, I. A. (1973). Some observations on the serology of *Pneumocystis carinii* infections in the United States. *Infect. Immunol.* **8**:317-321.

Nowoslawski, A., and Brzosko, W. J. (1964). Indirect immunofluorescence test for serodiagnosis of *Pneumocystis carinii* infection. *Bull. Acad. Polon. Sci.* **12**:143-147.

Pifer, L. L., Hughes, W. T., and Murphy, M. J., Jr. (1977). Propagation of *Pneumocystis carinii* in vitro. *Paediatr. Res.* **11**:305-316.

Pifer, L. L., Hughes, W. T., Stagno, S., and Woods, D. (1978). *Pneumocystis carinii* infection: Evidence for high prevalence in normal and immunosuppressed children. *Paediatrics* **61**:35-41.

Pintozzi, R. L. (1978). Morphological and immunological studies of experimentally propagated *Pneumocystis carinii*. Ph.D. dissertation, University of Illinois, Chicago.

Shepherd, V., Jameson, B., and Knowles, G. K. (1979). *Pneumocystis carinii* pneumonitis: A serological study. *J. Clin. Pathol.* **32**:773-777.

5

In Vitro Cultivation of *Pneumocystis*

JAMES W. SMITH and MARILYN S. BARTLETT

Indiana University School of Medicine
Indianapolis, Indiana

I. Historical Perspective

Culture of *Pneumocystis carinii* has been attempted by numerous workers since it was first recognized to be a pathogen. It has been variously considered to be a product of cell destruction, a virus, a fungus, and a protozoan (Goetz, 1960). Depending upon the view of workers as to its taxonomic position, various culture methods have been attempted. Goetz (1960) reviewed early culture studies stating that Pleiss attempted culture using a wide variety of bacteriologic media and reported that all attempts were unsuccessful.

Workers who considered *P. carinii* a fungus used media employed for cultivation of fungi. Several workers reported successful cultivation of *P. carinii* and proposed various fungal identifications. Csillag and Brandstein (1954-1955) reported successful cultivation of a fungus using Sabouraud's agar and malt agar. When inoculated into suckling mice, *Pneumocystis*-like structures were noted. They concluded that there were both vegetative forms and asci-containing ascopores, and that it was the latter which were found in the alveoli of infected humans and animals. Giese (1953a, b) also reported successful cultivation with fungus media and described the isolate as an ascomycetous fungus. Bauch and Ladstaetter (1953), using beer agar, cultivated a yeast from homogenates of lungs of 9 infants who died of interstitial plasma cell pneumonia. The isolate exhibited the forms seen in lung tissue only when streptomycin and penicillin were added to the medium. Bienengraber (1953, 1954) isolated *Candida pseudotropicalis* from lung tissue of children who had died of plasma cell pneumonia and also observed that after addition of penicillin to the growth medium, forms resembling *P. carinii* were present. He suggested that these forms either represented a stage of *C. pseudotropicalis* or *P. carinii* which were symbiotic with *C. pseudotropicalis* in the presence of penicillin. Other workers (Simon, 1953, 1955; Schmid, 1955), reported successful cultivation and identification of various fungi using agar media. A special yeast medium was employed by Stapka, et al. (1957) who isolated yeastlike organisms and reported that the addition of human serum induced intracellular structures in these organisms, but not the eight typical of *P. carinii* cysts. Jirovec (1954) and Jirovec and Vanek (1954), after reviewing the reported experiments, rejected the evidence that *P. carinii* was a fungus and that the cultivated organisms were *P. carinii.*

Jahn et al. (1957) inoculated embryonic chicken lung tissue cultures with homogenates of human lung obtained at autopsy and observed that in cultures with Hanks' balanced salt medium plus 10% horse serum, the organisms appeared unchanged for the first 8 days and after that there were signs of degeneration, so that by 22 days there was complete "dissolution." Gajdusek (1957) reported that embryonated hens' eggs had been used by Yugoslav workers in an unsuccessful attempt to culture organisms.

Recently, Pifer et al. (1977) attempted to propagate *P. carinii* in a variety of cell-free media which have been used for cultivation of a number of protozoa and fastidious bacteria, but were unsuccessful. Pesanti (1980) reports that the organisms can apparently remain viable in cell-free media for several days, but do not proliferate.

II. Recent Reports of Cultivation Attempts in Various Cell Lines

Renewed clinical interest in pneumocystosis, especially as it occurs in immunocompromised hosts, has resulted in increased interest in cultivation. Culture with varying degrees of success has been reported in four journal publications (Bartlett et al., 1979; Latorre et al., 1977; Pifer et al., 1977, 1978) from three groups, two doctoral dissertations (McManigal, 1979; Pintozzi, 1978a), and two recent abstracts (Cushion and Walzer, 1983; Sowar and Walzer, 1982). A wide variety of cell lines have been used and are summarized in Table 1. Some cell lines are only mentioned in the publications and some noted from our laboratory (Bartlett et al., unpublished) have not been reported.

Table 1 Cell Lines in Which Culture of *P. carinii* Has Been Attempted

Cell line	Pifer et al. (1978, 1979)	Latorre et al. (1977)	Bartlett et al. (1979)	McManigal (1979)	Pintozzi (1978a)	Sower and Walzer (1982)
WI-38 (Human embryonic lung fibroblast)	−		+	−	+	+[a]
CEL (Chick embryonic epithelial lung)	+			+	−	
Vero (African green monkey kidney)	+	+	+	+	+	
MRC-5 (Human embryo lung fibroblast)		+	+			
Chang (Human liver carcinoma)		+	+			
Secondary chicken embryo fibroblast	−					
Owl monkey kidney	+					
Baby hamster kidney	+					
AV-3 (Human amnion)	+					
LLC-MK2 (Rhesus monkey kidney)		−				
F1 (Human amnion)		−				
McCoy (Human synovium)		−				
AH-1 (African green monkey kidney)			+			
Rhesus monkey kidney				−		
HEp 2 (Human carcinoma of larynx)			−	−		
Fetal bovine kidney				+		
HeLa (Human carcinoma of cervix)				−		
LU-1 (Human lung carcinoma)					+	
MCF 7 (Human breast carcinoma)					+	
Walker (Rat carcinoma)			−			
A549 (Human lung carcinoma)			+			+
L2 (Adult rat lung)						+
RFL-6 (Fetal rat lung)						−
4/4 RM.4 (Rat visceral pleura)						−

[a]Cushion and Walzer (1983) also used a transformed WI-38 cell line.

Results of these studies differ, even for the same cell line, in part because of differences in methodology. A major difference is the means of evaluation of inocula and cultures. Some counted only cysts (McManigal, 1979; Pifer et al., 1977, 1978; Pintozzi, 197 8a) and others counted trophozoites (Bartlett et al., 1979; Sowar and Walzer, 1982). Means of obtaining organisms, sizes of inocula, stage(s) of organisms in inocula, incubation times, and techniques for transfer and harvest varied. In addition, the information presented does not always clearly explain experimental design and/or results.

In all studies, organisms for inocula were obtained from lungs of Sprague-Dawley rats treated with adrenal corticosteroids and tetracyclines as described by Frenkel et al. (1966). Such rats usually develop infection spontaneously due to activation of latent infection. Tetracycline is added to prevent bacterial infections. Organisms have generally been obtained from the lungs by agitation of incised lungs in liquid, or by crude homogenization. Only Pifer and co-workers (1977) have reported cultivation of organisms from infected human lung.

III. Morphologic Examination of Cultures

In order to better understand the culture studies, nomenclature of stages and methods of morphologic examination are briefly reviewed. Nomenclature of stages of the organism is not clearly defined because the taxonomy is not settled. Cysts have a cyst wall and variable numbers of intracystic organisms, up to eight in mature cysts. These intracystic organisms are variously called intracystic bodies or sporozoites. Organisms without a cyst wall are generally called trophozoites, although some call them thin-walled cysts. Stages in the transition between trophozoites and cysts are difficult to define. For practical purposes, cysts in these studies are organisms which stain with cyst wall stains.

Four principal methods may be used to examine cultures: stains which stain the cyst wall [methenamine silver nitrate, Gram-Weigert (Rosen et al., 1975), toluidine blue O (Chalvardjian and Graebe, 1963), and cresyl echt violet (Bowling et al., 1973)], stains which stain free trophozoites and intracystic organisms but do not stain the cyst wall (Giemsa, Wright's and polychrome methylene blue stains), phase contrast microscopy, and immunologic stains.

Other stains have been used to stain *P. carinii* in smears and/or sections and might be useful for cultures (Pintozzi et al., 1979; Ogino et al., 1977). These include Masson trichrome, Papanicolaou, periodic acid-Schiff (PAS), Gridley, Alcian blue, and Pappenheim stains.

Stains for the cyst wall are most widely used; however, such stains also stain fungal cell walls, and unless budding is seen, may not allow differentiation of fungi from *Pneumocystis* cysts (Reinhardt et al., 1977; Young et al., 1976). In addition, they will stain empty cysts, therefore, quantitative counts do not necessarily correlate with viable cysts. Routine methenamine silver stains take several hours to perform and have not been widely used on cultures, inocula, or tissue smears. Rapid methenamine silver stains have recently been described (Mahan and Sale, 1978; Pintozzi, 1978b; Semba, 1983) and were used in one study (Pintozzi, 1978a), but we have not had experience with them. Gram-Weigert stain is relatively easy to perform, but care must be taken to adequately decolorize in aniline-xylene so that background and cell nuclei are pink. There may be some irregularity of staining of some cysts so that only portions of the cysts are dark blue. In our experience, Gram-Weigert does not stain intracystic organisms although Pintozzi (1978a) states that they may be stained. Toluidine blue O is used by some investigators and appears to work well. We have not used this stain extensively. The cresyl echt violet (CEV) stain works quite well, although the organisms do not stain as darkly as with Gram-Weigert and methenamine silver stains, and so do not contrast as sharply with the background. The CEV stain requires glacial acetic acid and concentrated sulfuric acid, therefore, we do not use it routinely. Cyst stains are illustrated in Figure 1 (Gram-Weigert) and Figure 2 (methenamine silver nitrate and cresyl echt violet).

Giemsa stain in pH 7.0-7.2 phosphate buffer is a particularly useful stain, as it stains both free trophozoites and intracystic organisms. We use a 1:20 dilution of stock Giemsa in buffer and stain 30-40 min. There is some variance in stock Giemsa from various manufacturers and from lot to lot, so the ideal staining time must be determined with each new bottle of stock. Detection of cysts with 6-8 intracystic bodies is diagnostic of *P. carinii*, although cysts with fewer intracystic bodies may be recognized. The cyst wall may be seen as a negatively staining halo around the intracystic bodies. Free trophozoites in tissue smears or culture medium have a red nucleus and pale blue cytoplasm and usually appear in clumps. Giemsa stains are illustrated in Figures 3 and 4. We find it difficult to definitely identify trophozoites attached to culture cells. Trophozoites are difficult or impossible to recognize in homogenized tissue because of the large number of cell fragments. In impression smears of infected lung, cell fragments, especially those containing granules, may be difficult to differentiate from trophozoites. In tissue cultures, sloughed tissue culture cells and clumped trophozoites make it difficult to accurately count trophozoites. These are easier to count in medium from cell lines such as WI-38, in which fewer culture cells slough than in cell lines such as chick embryonic epithelial lung (CEL) and Chang liver in which sloughing is common. Cultures harvested by scraping the cells from the flask

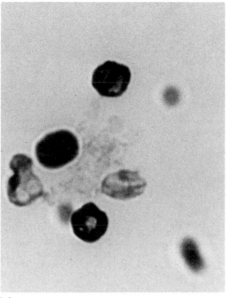

(a)

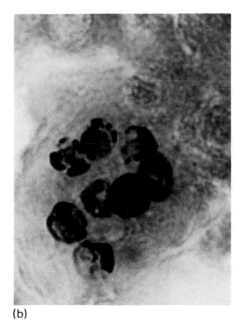

(b)

Figure 1 *P. carinii* cysts, Gram-Weigert, oil immersion. (a) *P. carinii* cysts from culture. There are also numerous trophozoites in the field, but they do not stain. (b) *P. carinii* cysts in an impression smear of infected lung. Note that there is variability in staining of most of the individual cysts, but one near the center stained uniformly.

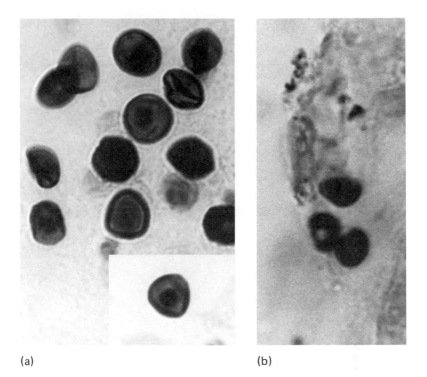

(a)   (b)

Figure 2 *P. carinii* cysts, impression smears of infected lungs, oil immersion. (a) Stained with methenamine silver nitrate and showing both rounded and irregular-shaped cysts. One organism has a darkly stained central area as is commonly seen in cysts. This is more clearly shown in the cysts in the insert. (b) Stained with cresyl echt violet and showing cysts with a similar appearance.

result in numerous cells and cell fragments, thus making it difficult to recognize trophozoites.

Phase contrast microscopy may be used to detect organisms in culture, but accurate quantitation is difficult. It does not work on ground material.

Specific immunologic stains may allow identification of *Pneumocystis* and specific immunofluorescent staining has been used on cultures (Pifer et al., 1977). In fluorescent antibody stains, neither cysts nor trophozoites show detailed morphology. Immunoperoxidase stain has been used to identify organisms (Bartlett and Smith, 1977; Levin et al., 1983) in tissue and impression smears but not in culture. Morphology of the cysts and trophozoites may be seen and the cyst walls are also stained.

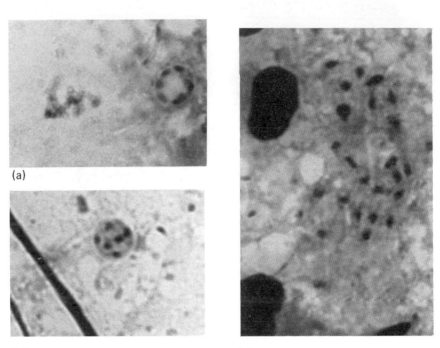

(a)

(b)   (c)

Figure 3 *P. carinii* cysts and trophozoites, lung impression smears, Giemsa stain, oil immersion. (a) and (b) Both show cysts. The upper cyst has the typical clock face distribution of the intracystic organisms, and the cyst wall is evident as a negatively staining halo surrounding the intracystic organism. Intracystic bodies in the lower cyst are distributed in a more irregular fashion and the cyst wall is not evident. A small clump of free trophozoites is evident to the left of the upper cyst. (c) A large number of free trophozoites. The large dark masses are tissue cell nuclei.

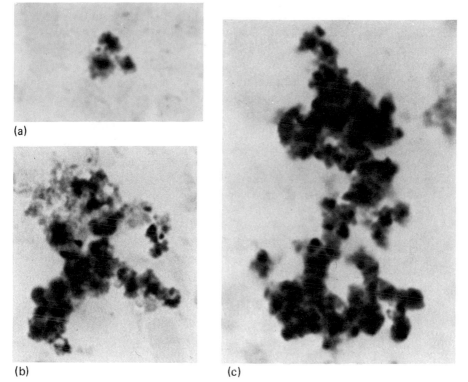

(a)

(b)

(c)

Figure 4 *P. carinii* trophozoites, WI-38 culture supernate, Giemsa stain, oil immersion. (a) A clump of three trophozoites in a 2-day culture. The clumps in (b) (4 days) and (c) (6 days) illustrate that clumps generally become larger with time. In some areas individual organisms may be seen.

IV. Culture Reports

The first report of cultivation of *P. carinii* was by Pifer et al. (1977). *Pneumocystis carinii* was propagated in chick embryonic epithelial lung cells (CEL). The CEL were 80-90% epithelial cells. Inocula for cultures were prepared from lungs of cortisone-treated Sprague-Dawley rats and from human lungs obtained at autopsy. The lung specimens were shaken in calcium and magnesium-free phosphate-buffered saline (CMF-PBS), the supernate centrifuged, and the pellets obtained, washed, and resuspended in medium 199 (M199). A sample of each inoculum was stained with toluidine blue O and examined microscopically. The number of cysts in each sample were counted. The coefficient of variation of the counting method was less than 2%. The number of trophozoites in the inoculum was not determined. Material was frozen at −15°C and checked to be sure there were no viable bacteria or fungi.

Each 24 hour CEL culture was inoculated with 9.1×10^4 cysts, 2.7×10^5 cysts, or with an inoculum containing trophozoites and very few cysts (less than 0.5% of the number of cysts in the original material). Medium was M199 with 10% fetal calf serum (FCS). Cultures were passed at 3 or 7 day intervals. The entire culture, that is culture cells and organisms, was used to inoculate new 24 hour CEL cultures. Some cultures were passed serially for four passages and others were split with each passage so that from an original culture there were 24 after four passages. Some cultures were harvested after three serial passages and *P. carinii* organisms separated by sucrose density gradients. Samples, 10 μl, were placed on slides, dried, fixed, and stored at −70°C for subsequent use in immunofluorescent staining.

When cultures of cells and organisms were serially passed in entirety to new cells, the number of cysts obtained after 4 passes at 3-day intervals was 2.3×10^7 for rat-derived *P. carinii.* The original inoculum was 2.7×10^5. This was an increase of approximately 10^2. Cultures derived from human sources were passed five times at 7-day intervals yielding 7.6×10^4 from an inoculum of 5×10^3. Cysts were both free in the medium and attached to cells. Serially passed cultures in which the inoculum was frozen before each passage showed a lower yield, suggesting that some organisms were killed by freezing and thawing.

When the CEL cultures were split with each passage, the total yield of cysts after 4 passages (24 cultures) was 1.5×10^6. The original inoculum was 9.1×10^4.

Cultures inoculated with trophozoites (0.5% cysts) yielded 2.8×10^3 cysts in the second passage; then the number decreased. Numbers of trophozoites in inoculum and culture were not determined.

In CEL, multiplication of organisms led to destruction of culture cells. Cytopathic effect (CPE) was noted within 24-74 hours after inoculation. Maximum CPE occurred with the greatest proliferation of organisms. CPE occurred in both the serially passed and the split-and-passed cultures. There was complete destruction of the monolayer when there was a ratio of 4 × 10^6 cysts to 2.4 × 10^7 cells. There was CPE in the cultures inoculated with trophozoites. If a light inoculum (less than 1 × 10^3 cysts/2.4 × 10^7 cells) was used, there was no detectable proliferation and no CPE. Cytopathic effect in CEL principally affected epithelial cells; fibroblasts appeared resistant to morphologic alteration.

Pifer noted that the most rapid increase in cyst numbers occurred in the first 24 hours and suggested that this was due to maturation to cysts of trophozoites in the inoculum.

Cultured organisms treated with fluorescein-labeled antibody to *P. carinii* fluoresced showing that the cysts from culture were indeed cysts of *P. carinii.* There was littel proliferation of cysts and little concomitant CPE of the monolayers when pentamidine isethionate or specific *P. carinii* antiserum was incorporated in the cultures. Inocula of autoclaved organisms from rat lung or culture showed no growth and no CPE.

Studies of life cycle, relationship of *P. carinii* to culture cells, and incorporation of ^{3}H-labeled thymidine, uridine, and amino acids were also performed and will be summarized later.

Latorre et al. (1977) described successful cultivation of *P. carinii* with 3 cell lines: Vero (African green monkey kidney), Chang liver (human liver carcinoma), and MRC-5 (human embryo lung fibroblast). Cell lines which did not support growth were LLC-MK2 (rhesus monkey kidney), FL (human amnion), and McCoy (human synovial fluid).

To prepare inocula, portions of infected lung from cortisone-treated Sprague-Dawley rats were ground in Eagle's minimal essential medium (MEM). The resulting homogenates were centrifuged at 500 *g* for 10-15 min. The first supernate was used for one inoculum. Additional resuspensions and centrifugations provided supernates for other inocula. Inocula were not quantitated for either cysts or trophozoites. Inoculum was added to well-developed monolayers in a ratio of 1 ml of inoculum to 5 ml of overlay. Medium for all cultures was MEM with 10% FCS.

Cultures were incubated at 37°C, and, after 4 days, clumps or organisms were observed in the culture flasks. Some clumps were floating in the media, and some appeared to be attached to the monolayers. To assure that the clumps were *P. carinii* organisms, both toluidine blue O and Giemsa stains were performed.

Inocula for subcultures were prepared in two ways, either medium containing organisms or medium containing organisms plus one-fourth of the monolayer scraped from the flask. In either case, the material was centrifuged and the resulting sediment resuspended in 1 ml of original medium.

One or the other of these inocula was used to inoculate fresh medium on new flasks. The sediment from one flask with 20 ml of medium was adequate to inoculate two more flasks containing 20 ml of medium plus one containing 5 ml of medium. Subculturing was done weekly for 4 months.

Vero, Chang liver, and MRC-5 supported growth. The yield of organisms was estimated to be an increase by at least a factor of 2 for each passage as determined by microscopic observation of the flasks. The 16 passages reported gave a theoretical total increase of 2^{16} or 65,536-fold. Both trophozoites and cysts were present in culture medium. Neither cysts nor trophozoites were counted, and the ratio of cysts to trophozoites was not reported. Clumps of organisms were first seen at 4 days and subcultures were performed at 7 days. No CPE was noted. Free-floating *Pneumocystis* removed by decanting medium from Vero and MRC-5 cell line cultures were free of monolayer cells. The medium decanted from Chang liver cultures did contain substrate cells.

Cultured organisms were used as antigen in an indirect immunofluorescent test.

Pifer et al. (1978), in a second publication, reported culture of *P. carinii* using Vero cell cultures. Other cell lines studied were owl monkey kidney, baby hamster kidney, AV-3 (human amnion), WI-38 (human embryonic lung fibroblasts), and secondary chicken embryo fibroblast cultures.

Inocula for cultures were prepared from lungs of cortisone-treated Sprague-Dawley rats. Portions of lung were shaken in CMF-PBS which was then centrifuged, and the resulting sediment resuspended in M199.

Twenty-four hour monolayers of cells were used for culture. Overlay media was discarded and the flasks were inoculated with 1-2 ml of media containing 1.3×10^5 to 8.5×10^5 cysts and incubated at 37°C for 2 hr. Additional fresh medium was then added to each flask and the cultures were incubated. Samples of 10 μl were removed daily, stained for cysts, and counted. A second method of quantitation was performed by scraping the monolayers from the flasks and combining the substrate cells with the overlay media and centrifuging before counting cysts.

In a second set of experiments using Vero cultures, after 24 hr, organisms were obtained from the overlay medium of one flask by centrifugation. They were then suspended in fresh medium and inoculated to a new flask. This was done serially for seven days. Fresh medium was also added to the original culture and both the "parent" and new culture were sampled daily for seven days for cyst counts. Two media were used, MEM with 2% FCS and M199 with 10% FCS.

Results of the first experiments showed a maximum increase of 10.8-fold at 72 hr and an increase of 3.6-fold in 24 hr in a culture with a cyst-to-cell ratio in the inoculum of 1:154. Yields with cyst-to-cell ratios of 1:28

and 1:278 were poorer and increased numbers were found only in first passages. With a ratio of 1:2778, there was no proliferation. There was moderate CPE with patchy sloughing of monolayers. Minimal essential medium with 2% FCS was superior to M199 with 10% FCS. Although they concluded that a cyst-to-cell ratio of 1:154 was best, they did not state the number of experiments performed at each ratio.

The second set of experiments was "only minimally successful," suggesting that frequent passages to fresh cells did not increase yield. No data were given.

Cultures in owl monkey kidney, baby hamster kidney, and AV-3 cell cultures showed approximately a threefold increase, and there was no growth in WI-38 and secondary chicken embryo fibroblast cultures.

Attempts to adapt the organisms to Vero cultures by passage of organisms at weekly or 3-day intervals for 12 weeks were described as unsuccessful after the third or fourth passage. Number of cysts decreased, trophozoites were rare, and there was diminished CPE, showing that there was no appreciable replication of organisms.

We (Bartlett et al., 1979) reported cultivation of *P. carinii* with WI-38 and MRC-5 cell cultures. In addition, Vero, Chang liver, and AH-1 cell lines were studied but not reported. The inocula for cultures were prepared by grinding portions of infected lung from cortisone-treated Sprague-Dawley rats in Eagle's MEM with 10% FCS. The homogenates were centrifuged at 150 g for 10 min and the supernates used as inocula. Because of difficulty in recognizing trophozoites in ground material, inocula were not quantitated. A 75 cm^2 flask containing 15 ml of overlay medium was inoculated with 1 ml of supernate.

Samples of medium were removed daily and trophozoites were quantitated in Giemsa-stained slides using the X 100 oil immersion objective. Clumping of trophozoites was a problem, but could be decreased by suspending organisms in medium free of divalent cations. The coefficient of variation of the counting method was approximately 15%.

When flasks were harvested by removal of all overlay medium and fresh medium was added, there was continued growth of *P. carinii*. This could be repeated a third time in some instances.

Subcultures were made by transferring 1 ml of overlay medium from a primary culture to a new monolayer with 15 ml of overlay medium. There was proliferation in two sequential subcultures, after which none could be demonstrated.

There was no destruction of the monolayers of WI-38, MRC-5 cells, Vero, or AH-1, and there was no CPE. The Chang liver monolayers were the only ones which showed significant sloughing of substrate cells. This was also reported by Latorre et al. (1977).

The amount of proliferation varied from culture to culture, and did not correlate well with the number of organisms observed in lungs used to prepare inocula. The inoculum from one rat proliferated so that a peak of 17.5×10^6 organisms was achieved. The time at which peak numbers of organisms were obtained varied, but in general was between the 4th and 8th day (Fig. 5). Few trophozoites could be found on the first or second day, and those which were detected were single or in pairs. After day 2, clumps of trophozoites were found and each day the clumps were larger so that by the peak day clumps were large and numerous. Often there were some cysts in the clumps, but the number varied with time and the particular culture.

Flasks of both WI-38 and MRC-5 cells in which proliferation had ceased were termed "used cells" and were reinoculated with infected rat lung. In one instance, they yielded as many organisms as new monolayers. Although used cells were kept with an overlay of maintenance medium for at least 2 weeks before being reused, it is possible that there were residual organisms on the substrate cells. The facts that CPE did not occur, monolayers could be reused, and that primary cultures could be replenished with new medium to produce a second harvest of organisms, show that the two fibroblast cell lines (WI-38 and MRC-5) were not greatly damaged by the organisms.

Differences in proliferation, using inocula from various rat lung specimens, were difficult to interpret. Some specimens may have contained other organisms such as viruses or mycoplasma which inhibited *P. carinii* proliferation. In addition, the ratios of cysts to trophozoites in the inocula may have differed but were not assessed.

Nutritional status of the rat appears to affect the ability of organisms to proliferate in culture. To hasten development of *Pneumocystis* infection in corticosteroid-treated rats, we placed some on a low-protein diet (Hughes et al., 1974). Organisms from lungs of these rats, although numerous, did not grow as well in WI-38 cultures as organisms from rats fed a normal diet.

The amount of proliferation in primary cultures was difficult to assess owing to the inability to accurately count trophozoites in the inoculum. The number of organisms counted in the overlay medium was not the total number in culture since some remained attached to substrate cells. Growth in MRC-5 cultures. The latter were more extensively studied because the cell line was readily available. We did not pursue Chang liver cultures because sloughed cells made counting difficult. There was some growth in Vero and AH-1 cell lines.

More recently we studied the effects of various oxygen concentrations on *Pneumocystis* cultures (Bartlett et al., 1983a), and have found that there is a greater yield in 5% O_2 plus 10% CO_2 than in gaseous mixtures with greater amounts of O_2 (12, 17, and 23%) plus 5-10% CO_2. Poorest yield was in ambient air. Reasons for the improved yield have yet to be defined,

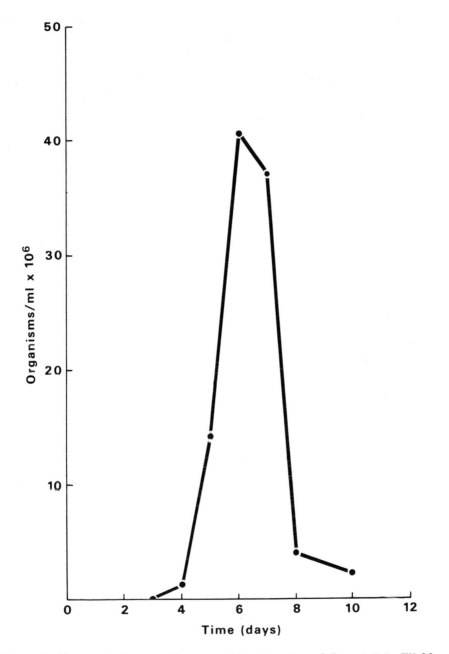

Figure 5 Representative growth curve of trophozoites of *P. carinii* in WI-38 cells. (From Bartlett et al., 1979.)

but possible explanations which might be important individually or in combination include (1) increased proliferation of *Pneumocystis* due to a direct effect on the organisms, (2) increased proliferation of *Pneumocystis* owing to a better substrate provided by WI-38 cells at lower O_2 tension, and (3) organisms survive better at lower O_2 tension. In spite of the improved yields at lowered O_2, continuous culture has not been achieved. We now perform all culture work in 5% O_2 plus 10% CO_2.

We have used cultured organisms in attempts to develop immunodiagnostic tests and to study phagocytosis by polymorphonuclear leukocytes. In addition, the culture system has been used to study scanning and transmission ultrastructure of *Pneumocystis* and antimicrobial susceptibility.

McMannigal (1979) attempted culture of *P. carinii* on the following cell lines: CEL, Vero, WI-38, rhesus monkey kidney, H.Ep-2 (human carcinoma of the larynx), HeLa (human carcinoma of the cervix), and fetal bovine kidney. The inoculum was obtained by agitation of lungs from corticosteroid-treated male Sprague-Dawley rats, and quantitated by toluidine blue O stains. Inocula varied from 1×10^5 to 4×10^5 cysts per 75 cm^2 flask containing 12 ml of medium. The most common inoculum was 2.6×10^5 cysts. Some inocula were frozen at $-70°C$ before use, but the author did not state which experiments used frozen inocula.

The CEL cultures were prepared by a method similar to that of Pifer et al. (1977). The proportion of culture cells that were epithelial was not stated. The average inoculum was 2.12×10^4/ml of medium. Flasks were harvested on the third day by scraping with a rubber policeman. Serial cultures were made by transferring the entire yield from one flask to a second CEL monolayer. McManigal does not state if more than one serial transfer was attempted or if there was CPE. She also evaluated the influence of the concentration of FCS, heat inactivation of FCS, and the influence of glucose and glucose plus insulin.

In CEL, she found an approximate doubling of the number of cysts on the initial culture with an additional doubling in one serial transfer; however, she could not obtain the tenfold yields described by Pifer.

Yields from cultures with 0 or 1% FCS were slightly higher ($2.5 \times$ inoculum) than with 10% FCS ($1.8 \times$ inoculum). There was no increase of *P. carinii* cysts with 20% FCS ($0.73 \times$ inoculum). Heat inactivation of FCS did not affect yield. With added glucose or glucose plus insulin there was no increase in the number of cysts.

Cultures in Vero cells were inoculated with 3.0×10^3 to 3.7×10^4/ml cysts and FCS varied from 0 to 20%. They were harvested after a minimum of three days and yield varied from $2.8 \times$ to $0.6 \times$ inoculum (average $1.4 \times$ inoculum). McManigal felt that the optimum inoculum ratio of cysts to cells was 1:150-1:200. She did not report any attempted transfers. She stated that Vero cells did not scrape from the flasks easily, and therefore, the harvests from these monolayers contained less host cell material.

WI-38, rhesus monkey kidney, H.Ep-2, and HeLa cell lines did not support cyst proliferation with either 0 or 10% FCS. Fetal bovine kidney yielded a twofold increase in *P. carinii* cysts.

In McManigal's studies, the number of trophozoites in inoculum and cultures was not evaluated and cultures were only held for 3-5 days. Because of poor yields with cultures, she abandoned them.

She did note that female Sprague-Dawley rats appeared to be more susceptible to *P. carinii* infection than male rats.

Pintozzi (1978a) also attempted to culture *P. carinii* obtained from lungs of corticosteroid-treated Sprague-Dawley rats. Inoculum was obtained by agitation or by hand grinding of infected lungs. The material for inoculation was stored at $4°C$. Cell lines used were CEL, Vero, WI-38, LU-1 (also called Calu-1, from human lung carcinoma), and MCF-7 (human breast carcinoma). Numbers of cysts in inocula and cultures were determined in toluidine blue O or Gomori's methenamine silver nitrate stains. Numbers of trophozoites were not determined. Inocula were 10^5-10^6 cysts per ml except for WI-38, which received an inoculum of 10^4-10^5 cysts per ml. Cultures were harvested in 3-7 days.

The CEL was prepared from 14-day chick embryos and medium contained 10% FCS, but had only 50% epithelial cells in contrast to 80-90% in Pifer's study. Inoculum was obtained by agitation of infected rat lung in CMF-PBS. He could not demonstrate proliferation of *P. carinii* in this cell line and suggested that this may have been because of the low percentage of epithelial cells.

Vero cell line inoculated with hand-ground infected lung showed some proliferation ($1.6 \times$ inoculum to $4.0 \times$ inoculum) by three days, but cells sloughed in 48-72 hours; subculture was unsuccessful. In most cultures of WI-38 inoculated with lung homogenate, there was no proliferation, but some yielded 2.2-$3.5 \times$ inoculum at three days. LU-1 yielded $1.3 \times$ inoculum by the third day, at which time the cells sloughed. Subculture was unsuccessful.

Best results were obtained with MCF-7 which showed a 10-20-fold increase in the number of cysts by the third day. Unfortunately, culture in this cell line was not pursued further. Pintozzi does note that for this cell line, medium was changed 24 hr after inoculation and he feels that this may have contributed to the increased cyst counts.

He used cultured organisms for histochemical and immunologic studies, but is not clear concerning which of the studies were performed on cultured organisms and which were performed on organisms obtained from rat lungs.

Sowar and Walzer (1982) studied proliferation of *Pneumocystis* in a variety of cell lines. Quantitation was performed by (1) counting trophozoites in Giemsa stain and cysts in crseyl echt violet stain and (2) examining total flask contents for supernatant and cell-associated cysts. They found that in all cell lines, cyst counts declined on days 1-2, increased on days 3-6, and fell after day 7. There were more cysts in supernatant than in the monolayer fraction. Trophozoite counts were tenfold greater than cyst counts. Greatest proliferation (up to 10X) was found with A549 (human lung carcinoma), intermediate with WI-38, and L2 (adult rat lung), and least with RFL-6 (rat fetal lung) and 4/4 RM.4 (rat visceral pleura).

Very recently Cushion and Walzer (1983) further studied *Pneumocystis* culture in A-549 and in WI-38 VA13 subline 2RA. The latter is an SV40 transformed WI-38 cell line. Inoculum was from corticosteroid-treated rats. An inoculum of 10^5-10^6 *Pneumocystis* was needed to establish growth, and a 5-10-fold increase in numbers of organisms was achieved over a two-week period. *Pneumocystis* could be passed three additional times in A549 cell line but not in the transformed WI-38 cell line. Three factors were noted to enhance growth: 20% fetal calf serum was better than other concentrations tested, stationary cultures grew better than cultures on a shaker, and organisms grew better in closed flasks than in a 5% CO_2 atmosphere. One of ten cultures of *Pneumocystis* from infected human lung showed a tenfold increase over two weeks in A549, but the other nine did not show proliferation.

V. Discussion of Culture Systems

All authors used *Pneumocystis* organisms obtained from Sprague-Dawley rats which had been treated with corticosteroids for an extended period of time. McManigal (1979) suggested that female rats may more readily develop *pneumocystis* infection than males, and thus may be preferred. She also noted that subcutaneous steroid injections were more reliable than giving the drug in water because the amount of liquid consumed by the rats varied. We attempted to accelerate development and severity of infection by giving a low-protein diet in addition to the steroid therapy, and found that the *Pneumocystis* organisms from these rats grew less well in culture. *Pneumocystis* from infected human lung has not been reproducibly cultured. Pifer et al. (1977) reported the only successful culture of *Pneumocystis* from infected human lung. We have attempted culture from infected human lung on a number of occasions, but have not shown reproducible proliferation comparable to that noted from infected rat lung.

Before preparing inocula, impression smears of the lung should be stained to be sure there are no bacteria or fungi because antibiotics incorporated in the medium may not always suppress these organisms. Inoculum may still contain viruses, mycoplasma, or other organisms not detected in smears, and this may explain poorer yields from cultures of lungs of some rats.

Lungs were variously processed by incising, then agitating in CMF-PBS, or by grinding in tissue grinders. Pifer and co-workers (1977) routinely froze inocula while checking for sterility, and McManigal (1979) sometimes froze inocula. Both reported successful cultivation of organisms from frozen inocula.

We have also found that frozen rat lung provides a satisfactory source of inoculum (unpublished observations) after storage for up to 6 months at -70°C. Fresh lung or lung which has been frozen for a short period provides a somewhat greater yield. Use of frozen lung has been a major improvement for culture systems, as freshly sacrificed infected rats are not required to provide inoculum each time a culture is done.

The size of inoculum required is not well defined. With very small inocula, growth has not been obtained, suggesting that a critical number of organisms may be required to establish infection. The ratio of organisms to cells may be important as suggested by data from Pifer et al. (1977, 1978) and McManigal (1979). In Vero cells, Pifer found maximum proliferation with a ratio of 1 cyst per 154 cells, and McManigal with 1 cyst per 150-200 cells. Trophozoites were not counted in their inocula. Proportions of cysts and trophozoites in infected lungs vary, and the role of trophozoites in cyst proliferation and vice versa is not yet defined. Ideally, the number of cysts and trophozoites and the ratios of each to culture cells should be determined for inocula. Optimal ratios for various cell lines may differ.

Media used in the various studies were either M199 or Eagle's MEM with varied amounts of FCS. McManigal (1979) suggested that cyst proliferation in Vero cells may be better if there is little or no FCS. Pifer et al. (1978) showed that there was better cyst proliferation in Vero cells using MEM with 2% FCS than using M199 with 10% FCS. McManigal (1979) also noted that heat inactivation of the FCS did not affect cyst proliferation, suggesting that complement was not inhibitory. We suggest that lower amounts of FCS may provide a less nutritious medium, thus stimulating cyst formation, or conversely that FCS may in some way inhibit cyst formation. Studies in which both cyst and trophozoite proliferation are evaluated in varying concentration of FCS may elucidate the role of FCS in cultures.

In general, only cysts have been counted in cultures although trophozoites were occasionally looked for by Pifer's group (1977, 1978) and have been the principal organisms counted by Bartlett et al. (1979). An ideal system would allow enumeration of both cysts and trophozoites in inocula and cultures, both cell-associated and free in medium. Perhaps use of immunological stains such as immunoperoxidase or immunofluorescence would be helpful, especially if antisera specific for cysts and antisera specific for trophozoites were used. Ikai (1980) has recently reported development of trophozoite-specific and cyst wall-specific antibody. In IFA, his trophozoite antibody stains trophozoites and intracystic bodies but not cyst walls, and his cyst antibody stains cyst walls. These reagents have not been used on cultured organisms.

A wide variety of cell lines have been used, but for most there is little published data. Those best described are Vero, CEL, WI-38, MRC 5, and Chang liver. Some cell lines may be better for cysts and others better for trophozoites. In addition, time of incubation is important. For example, Pifer et al. (1978) noted maximum proliferation of cysts in the first 24 hr in Vero. We (Bartlett et al., 1979) have used Giemsa-stained smears for counting, and count both trophozoites and cysts, but in our system trophozoites predominate until quite late. We have noted maximum numbers of organisms in approximately 6 days in WI-38 monolayers. Numbers of cysts increased with time so that a three-week culture showed a preponderance of cysts.

Cytopathic effect (CPE) was noted in CEL by all authors who studied this system, and was noted in Vero by Pifer et al. (1978) and Pintozzi (1978a), but not by Bartlett et al. (1979) or Latorre et al. (1977). McManigal (1979) does not comment on whether there was CPE in the Vero cell line.

Most authors noted that growth was limited generally to a maximum of 4 passages, although Latorre reported achieving 16 passages. Our studies suggest that a factor in the inoculum is depleted, but they have not been repeated systematically since we began cultivating in 5% O_2 plus 10% CO_2 (Bartlett et al., 1983a). Further studies of culture systems are needed with the goals of achieving continuous culture, producing large numbers of cysts and/or trophozoites, and reproducibly growing *Pneumocystis* from infected human lung.

VI. Uses of Cultured Organisms

A variety of studies have been performed using culture systems or organisms grown in the culture systems.

Two groups, Pifer et al. (1977) and Murphy et al. (1977), have studied the life cycle and morphology of cultured organisms. The Pifer group, using phase contrast microscopy, studied the growth of organisms in CEL in a Sykes-Moore chamber. They reported that the reproductive cycle took 4-6 hr. Trophozoites attached to cells loosely by strandlike fibers in approximately 30 min and then became somewhat smaller. After 90 min of attachment, organisms detached and became rounded, developing into cysts. Intra-

cystic organisms were evident 4 hr postinoculation and the number of intracystic organisms increased. Excystment occurred at single or multiple sites
and the newly excysted organisms (trophozoites) then became attached to
cells in 30-120 min. Cysts sometimes remained dormant. Trophozoite division was not observed.

Our studies suggest that trophozoites can divide, as we saw very few
cysts in our material during the period of rapid proliferation, although this
is admittedly circumstantial. It is also possible that trophozoites may be
able to divide in some cell cultures but not in others.

Morphology of cultured organisms by scanning electron microscopy
(SEM), reported by Murphy et al. (1977), has shown that organisms are outside the culture cells and produce three kinds of fibrils. One type of fibril
appears to attach the parasite to the host cell. A second type of fibril inter-
connects parasites and may allow materials to be exchanged between organisms. A third type of fibril with a hollow core anastomoses with the plasma-
lemma of the host cell and is hypothesized to transfer nutrients. They noted
an amorphous matrix containing membranes associated with aggregates of
Pneumocystis, but could not determine the origin of this matrix. Buds pro-
truding from occasional cysts were interpreted to be intracystic organisms
which were escaping. Cup-shaped cysts, similar to those noted by light
microscopy with cyst wall stains, were interpreted as representing cysts from
which the intracystic organisms had escaped. Rounded cysts had many
microvilli on their surfaces, whereas cup-shaped cysts were smoother.

Hull, working with us, has not demonstrated these various types of
fibrils by SEM in the WI-38 culture system. Transmission electron microscopy (TEM) of clumps of *Pneumocystis* trophozoites in matrix suggest that
the matrix is composed of cell membrane material derived from the organisms.

In addition, Hull et al. (1983a) have studied cell wall and cell membrane
glycoproteins in cultured *Pneumocystis* stained-fixed in Ruthenium red-osmium.
Walls of cysts, trophozoites, and psuedopodia contained acidic glycoproteins.
Cyst walls contained four layers, whereas trophozoite walls contained two
layers. Trophozoite pseudopodia appeared to be outpouchings of the entire
trophozoite wall. In cysts, the pseudopodia had two layers continuous with
the outer two layers of cyst wall but not the inner two.

Pifer et al. (1977) also studied the metabolism of organisms in CEL
culture by autoradiographic methods using [³H] thymidine, [³H] uridine, and
³H-labeled amino acids in separate experiments. Labeled substances were incorporated in media and the CEL cultures incubated for 48 hr. The cultures
were then rinsed and inoculated with *P. carinii* cysts. After an additional
48 hr, cultures were examined by autoradiographic methods for incorporation
of label into cysts. Results showed that the labeled amino acids were distributed throughout the cysts, uridine was present throughout the cysts but

was concentrated near the periphery and thymidine was concentrated in clearly demarcated foci at the periphery of the cysts corresponding to the location of the intracystic organisms. They conclude that materials derived from CEL cells are incorporated into the proteins, RNA, and DNA of the *Pneumocystis.*

Cultured organisms have been used for immunodiagnostic tests. Pifer et al. (1977) mention that cultured organisms for IFA tests and organisms grown by Latorre's group (Latorre et al., 1977) have been used for IFA serologic tests at the Centers for Disease Control. Latorre noted that although organisms from MRC-5 and Vero cell lines gave good results, he preferred the organisms from Chang liver culture because sloughed substrate cells provided a contrasting background. Pifer has immunized animals with cultured organisms and used the antibody in a counterimmunoelectrophoresis test to detect pneumocystis antigen.

With another group we have studied phagocytosis of cultured *Pneumocystis* trophozoites by polymorphonuclear leukocytes (Oseas et al., 1979). We found that *Pneumocystis* are readily phagocytized if antibody is present, but are not readily phagocytized when antibody is not present.

Recently, antimicrobial susceptibility of *Pneumocystis* in culture has been studied by members of our group (Bartlett et al., 1983b; Smith et al., 1983) and by Pifer et al. (1983) using different methods.

Early studies in our laboratory (Smith et al., 1983) looked at three different ways of using our culture system. One added drug to primary culture at the same time that infected rat lung was inoculated to the culture. The second used outgrowth cultures. Supernatant of primary cultures was harvested, then new medium containing drug was added. (Previous work showed that many *Pneumocystis* organisms were still attached to WI-38 cells). The third was subcultures in which a supernatant of an infected culture was inoculated to new WI-38 cells at the same time drug was added. In all instances counts were performed on aliquots of culture supernatants. All were incubated in 5% O_2 and 20% CO_2 at 35°C. The results showed marked inhibition of *Pneumocystis* by 10 μg/ml of pentamidine with slight inhibition by trimethoprim-sulfamethoxazole (TMP/SMX) 50:200 μg/ml. The results were more clear cut and the method more reproducible using outgrowth cultures, so subsequent studies (Bartlett et al., 1983) have used this system. A number of drugs were studied and in this system, *Pneumocystis carinii* was inhibited by pentamidine isethionate (0.5 and 5 μg/ml), TMP-SMX (50:200 μg/ml), miconazole (2 and 20 μg/ml), chloroquine (2 and 20 μg/ml), and high concentrations of amphotericin B (5 μg/ml). *Pneumocystis* were not inhibited by low concentrations of amphotericin B (0.5 μg/ml) or metronidazole (2 and 10 μg/ml). Representative growth curves are shown in Figure 6.

With the above method, organisms attached to monolayers are not counted, only supernatant organisms. In some instances we have looked at organisms on monolayers by having glass coverslips in wells when WI-38 cells are added. The cells then sheet out on the coverslips and later can be removed and stained to assess numbers of cell-associated organisms. Unfortunately, there is often granular debris of stain precipitate which may be difficult to differentiate from trophozoites. Another potential problem is that our counting system does not differentiate viable from nonviable organisms.

Hull, of our group, has performed SEM of *Pneumocystis* exposed to pentamidine isethionate or TMP-SMX (Hull et al., 1983b) in the above culture system. *Pneumocystis* trophozoites which had not been exposed to antimicrobials showed numerous complex surface pseudopodia. Trophozoites exposed to pentamidine showed progressively fewer and shorter pseudopodia from days 1-7. At day 3, trophozoites had prominent suface blebs which often became detached. Trimethoprim-sulfamethoxazole treated trophozoites also showed fewer pseudopodia than controls.

Pifer and colleagues (1983) recently reported a culture system to assess antimicrobial susceptibility of *Pneumocystis* from infected rat lung using CEL. In this system, cysts were counted in culture supernate, and cell-associated cysts were determined by examining coverslips covered by monolayers. Numbers of cysts increased markedly in the first 24 hr, both cell associated and free in supernatants. Numbers of cysts showed minimal increase in the presence of TMP-SMX or pentamidine. After exposure to antimicrobials, cysts were washed and inoculated to new cells, but did not proliferate.

Future studies of susceptibility should attempt to enumerate both cysts and trophozoites which are both cell associated and free. Assessment of viability is also needed.

Smith and Bartlett, working with D. Moss and H. Mathews at the Centers for Disease Control, attempted to look at isoenzymes of *Pneumocystis* from the rat model cultured on WI-38 cells. Soluble material for the studies was prepared by sonicating a washed harvest of *Pneumocystis* which generally contained less than 1% WI-38 cells and 10^7-10^8 *Pneumocystis* trophozoites per milliliter. These preliminary studies showed that *Pneumocystis* has isoenzymes which can be detected. The goal was to compare isoenzyme patterns of rat and human *Pneumocystis* to see if there were differences. Unfortunately, adequate numbers of sufficiently pure *Pneumocystis* from infected humans could not be obtained.

To our knowledge, the above are the only studies using cultured organisms.

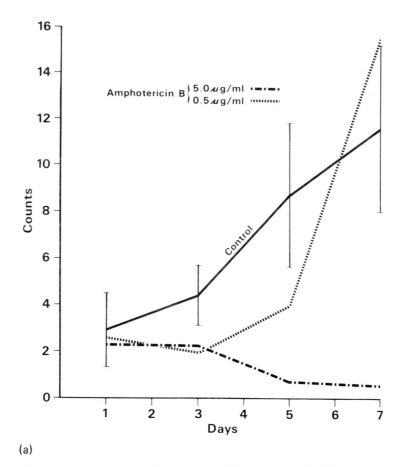

(a)

Figure 6 Representative growth curves in the presence of (a) amphotericin B and (b) pentamidine isethionate.

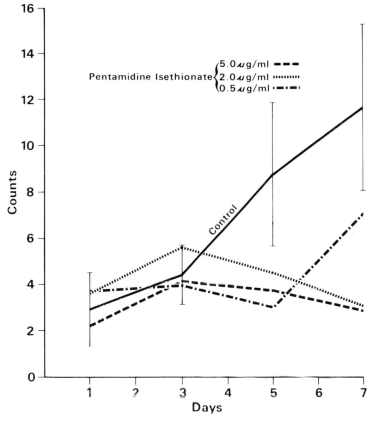

(b)

Figure 6 (continued)

VII. Future Uses of Cultured Organisms

Pneumocystis from infected rat lungs can now be grown reproducibly and in reasonable quantities. It is hoped that *Pneumocystis* from infected human lungs will soon be cultured as successfully. Cultured organisms and culture systems can be used to study taxonomy, biology, structure, antimicrobial susceptibility, and pathogenesis.

The life cycle of the organism must be better defined. The relative importance of cysts and trophozoites in proliferation must be clarified and the stimuli which lead to encystment and excystment defined. The structure and method of formation of cyst walls needs to be elucidated. Culture offers the opportunity to study these processes using techniques such as metabolic inhibitors, immunologic markers, isotopic labels, to name a few.

Organism-cell interaction should be studied in more detail to elucidate the role of cells in growth and proliferation of organisms and to learn how organisms damage cells in cell lines in which damage has been demonstrated.

Matrix which surrounds clumps of organisms in infected human lung is proposed to contain residual host cell material and immunoglobulins (Brzosko et al., 1976). In culture, clumping of organisms with matrix was observed and Murphy et al. (1977), who suggest that the matrix contains membranes, possibly of host cell origin. In our studies using WI-38 cultures, no CPE was noted, suggesting that the matrix was not derived from culture cells, and, as mentioned above, we feel that matrix resembles *Pneumocystis* cell membrane material. Further studies are needed.

Cultured organisms may answer a number of questions about the epidemiology and pathogenesis of pneumocystis infection. Are cysts, trophozoites, or both cysts and trophozoites infective and how long do they remain viable in the environment? Are there other forms? What are the roles of cell-mediated immunity and humoral immunity in host defenses? What factors are necessary for effective phagocytosis and subsequent destruction of organisms by both polymorphonuclear leukocytes and macrophages? What are the roles of trophozoites versus cysts in the development of clinical disease?

In addition to studying antimicrobial susceptibility of *Pneumocystis* in cultures, cultivated organisms can be used as a source of enzymes for in vitro susceptibility testing. For example, dihydrofolate reductase could be purified from cultured *Pneumocystis,* and its susceptibility to various analogues of pentamidine could be studied. With Queener we have performed preliminary studies which show promise in this area (Queener et al., 1984). In addition, studies of susceptibility in vitro, in cell culture, and in animal models can be correlated to better understand mechanisms of action of drugs.

Improved culture systems should provide better sources of antigen. This could allow studies of antigen variability among strains of *pneumocystis* and could clarify the relationship or organisms causing rat and human infections. Better antigen could lead to development of more sensitive and more specific immunodiagnostic tests. More reliable tests for antigen detection would be particularly helpful.

Lastly, cultured organisms could provide a source of relatively pure pneumocystis DNA for studies of the molecular biology of the organism.

VIII. Summary

Cultivation of *P. carinii* in cell cultures has had limited use to date. Yields have been poor but are improving. Most studies have had four or less successful passages. Although inocula for all studies have included both cysts and trophozoites, most authors have emphasized quantitation of cysts (McManigal, 1979; Pifer et al., 1977, 1978; Pintozzi, 1978a), whereas we (Bartlett et al., 1979) have emphasized trophozoites but have also counted cysts. Different cell lines have given different results. Chick embryonic epithelial lung cells have shown CPE, whereas WI-38 and MRC-5 have not. There is disagreement on CPE with Vero cells. Time for development of cysts is relatively short for CEL but longer for WI-38 and MRC-5. Increasing amounts of FCS in the medium appears to decrease the yield of cysts in Vero cells (McManigal, 1979; Pifer et al., 1978). Results with WI-38 and MRC-5 suggest that a factor or factors in the inoculum become depleted with time. It is hoped that these factors can be discovered and used to develop better culture systems. Recent use of cultured *Pneumocystis* for studies of morphology, biochemistry, immunology, and antimicrobial susceptibility suggests that culture systems will be crucial for a better understanding of *Pneumocystis* and for improving diagnosis and therapy.

References

Bartlett, M. S., and Smith, J. W. (1977). Identification of *Pneumocystis carinii* by immunoperoxidase staining. Abstracts of the Annual Meeting of the American Society for Microbiology, New Orleans, Louisiana. American Society for Microbiology, Washington, D.C., page 37.

Bartlett, M. S., Verbanac, P. A., and Smith, J. W. (1979). Cultivation of *Pneumocystis carinii* with WI-38 cells. *J. Clin. Microbiol.* **10**:796-799.

Bartlett, M. S., Eichholtz, R., Miller, J., and Smith, J. W. (1983a). Enhanced in vitro proliferation of *Pneumocystis carinii* with lowered O levels. Abstracts of the Annual Meeting of the American Society for Microbiology, New Orleans, Louisiana. American Society for Microbiology, Washington, D.C., page 66.

Bartlett, M. S., Eichholtz, R., Miller, J., and Smith, J. W. (1983b). Activity of antimicrobial agents against *Pneumocystis carinii* in culture. Abstracts of the Interscience Conference on Antimicrobial Agents and Chemotherapy, Las Vegas, Nevada. American Society for Microbiology, Washington, D.C., page 173.

Bauch, R., and Ladstaetter, L. *Pneumocystis carinii* and interstitial plasma cell pneumonia in premature infant. *Klin. Woehenschr.* 31:900-903.

Bienengraber, A. (1953). Beitrag zar Enzephalitis bei fruhkindlicher interstitieller pneumonie. *Aentralbl. Allg. Pathol.* 89:287-288.

Bienengraber, A. (1954). Zür Frage der atiologeschen Bedeutung der Kandidazeen bei interstitieller plasmazellularer pneumonie. *Zentralbl. Allg. Pathol.* 92:225-227.

Bowling, M. C., Smith, I. M., and Wescott, S. L. (1973). A rapid staining procedure for *Pneumocystis carinii. Am. J. Med. Technol.* 39:267-268.

Brzosko, W. J., Krawcynski, K., Madalinski, K., and Nowoslawski, A. (1976). Immunopathologic aspects of *Pneumocystis carinii* pneumonia in infants as revealed by immunofluorescence and electron microscopy. Symposium on *Pneumocystis carinii* infection. Washington, D. C., DHEW Pub. No. 76-90 (NIH). 163-169.

Chalvardjian, A. W., and Graebe, L. A. (1963). A new procedure for the identification of *Pneumocystis carinii* cysts in tissue sections and smears. *J. Clin. Pathol.* 16:383-385.

Csillag, A., and Brandstein, L. (1954-1955). The role of a Blastomyces in the aetiology of interstitial plasmocytic pneumonia of the premature infant. *Acta Microbiol. Hung.* 1-2:179-190.

Cushion, M. T., and Walzer, P. D. (1983). Conditions for *In Vitro Pneumocystis carinii* culture using two human lung derived cell lines. American Society of Parasitologists, San Antonio (Abstract 146).

Frenkel, J. K., Good, J. T., and Schultz, J. A. (1966). Latent *Pneumocystis* infection in rats, relapse and chemotherapy. *Lab. Invest.* 15:1559-1577.

Gajdusek, D. C. (1957). *Pneumocystis carinii*–etiologic agent of interstitial plasma cell pneumonia of premature and young infants. *Pediatrics* 19:543-565.

Giese, W. (1953a). Etiology of the interstitial plasmacellular infant pneumonia. *Monatsschr. Kinderheilkd* 101:147-149.

Giese, W. (1953b). Pathogenese und atiologie der interstitiellen plasmagellularen sauglines pneumonie. *Zentralbl. Allg. Pathol.* 90:54.

Goetz, O. (1960). Dic atiologie der interstitiellen sagenannten plasmagellularen pneumonie des jugen sanglins. *Archiv. Kinderheilkd* 161:41:1.

Hughes, W. T., Price, R. A., Sisko, F., Havron, W. S., Kafatos, A. G., Schonland, M., and Smythe, P. M. (1974). Protein-calorie malnutrition a host determinant for *Pneumocystis carinii* infection. *Am. J. Dis. Child.* **128**:44-52.

Hull, M. T., Bartlett, M. S., Goheen, M. P., and Smith, J. W. (1983a). Electron microscopic study of cell wall glycoproteins in *Pneumocystis carinii* in vitro and in vivo. *Lab. Invest.* **48**:6P.

Hull, M. T., Bartlett, M. S., Goheen, M. P., and Smith, J. W. (1983b). Effects of pentamidine isethionate on cultured *Pneumocystis carinii:* A scanning electron microscopic study. Abstracts of the Annual Meeting of the American Society for Microbiology, New Orleans, Louisiana. American Society for Microbiology, Washington, D.C., page 20.

Ikai, T. (1980). *Pneumocystis carinii:* Production of antibody either specific to trophozoite or to cyst wall. *Jpn. J. Parasitol.* **29**:115-126.

Jahn, E., and Roller-Gusende, R. E. (1957). Serology and clinical aspects of interstitial plasma cell pneumonia. *Klin. Wochenschr.* **35**:37-41.

Jirovec, O. (1954). Interstitial pneumonia in infants caused by *Pneumocystis carinii. Monatsschr. Kinderheilkd* **102**:476-485.

Jirovec, O., and Vanek, J. (1954). Morphology of *Pneumocystis carinii* and pathogenesis of *Pneumocystis carinii* pneumonia. *Zentralbl. Allg. Pathol.* **92**:424-437.

Latorre, C. R., Sulzer, A. J., and Norman, L. G. (1977). Serial propagation of *Pneumocystis carinii* in cell line cultures. *Appl. Environ. Microbiol.* **33**:1204-1206.

Levin, M., McLeod, R., Young, Q., Abrahams, C., Chambliss, M., Walzer, P., and Kabins, S. A. (1983). *Pneumocystis* pneumonia: Importance of gallium scan in early diagnosis and description of a new immunoperoxidase technique to demonstrate *Pneumocystis carinii. Am. Rev. Respir. Dis.* **128**:182-185.

Mahan, C. T., and Sale, G. E. (1978). Rapid methenamine silver stain for *Pneumocystis* and fungi. *Arch. Pathol. Lab. Med.* **102**:351-352.

McManigal, S. A. N. (1979). Pneumocystosis: Host-parasite relationships. Ph.D. dissertation, University of Oklahoma Health Sciences Center, Oklahoma City.

Murphy, M. J., Pifer, L. L., and Hughes, W. T. (1977). *Pneumocystis carinii* in vitro—a study by scanning electron microscopy. *Am. J. Pathol.* **86**:387-394.

Ogino, K., Yoshida, Y., Takeuchi, S., Ikai, T., and Yamada, M. (1977). Studies on *Pneumocystis carinii* and *Pneumocystis carinii* pneumonia I. Evaluation of several kinds of staining methods in the identification of *P. carinii. Jpn. J. Parasitol.* **26**:116-126.

Oseas, R. S., Bartlett, M. S., Baehner, R. L., Boxer, L. A., and Smith, J. W. (1979). *Pneumocystis carinii* trophozoites require opsonization for phagocytosis by polymorphonuclear leukocytes. *Fed. Proc. (Abstr. 4084)* **38**:1002.

Pesanti, E. L. (1980). In vitro effects of antiprotozoan drugs and immune serum on *Pneumocystis carinii. J. Infect. Dis.* **141**(6):775-780.

Pifer, L. L., Hughes, W. T., and Murphy, M. J. (1977). Propagation of *Pneumocystis carinii* in vitro. *Pediatr. Res.* **11**:305-316.

Pifer, L. L., Woods, D., and Hughes, W. T. (1978). Propagation of *Pneumocystis carinii* in vero cell culture. *Infect. Immun.* **20**:66-68.

Pifer, L. L., Pifer, D. D., and Woods, D. R. (1983). Biological profile and response to anti-pneumocystis agents of *Pneumocystis carinii* in cell culture. *Antimicrob. Agents Chemother.* **24**:674-678.

Pintozzi, R. L. (1978a). Morphological and immunological studies of experimentally propagated *Pneumocystis carinii.* Ph.D. dissertation, University of Illinois, Chicago.

Pintozzi, R. L. (1978b). Technical methods-modified Grocott's methenamine silver nitrate method for quick staining of *Pneumocystis carinii. J. Clin. Pathol.* **31**:803-805.

Pintozzi, R. L., Blecka, L. J., and Nanos, S. (1979). The morphologic identification of *Pneumocystis carinii. Acta Cytol.* **23**:35-39.

Queener, S. F., Gettinger, P., Bartlett, M., and Smith, J. W. (1984). Sensitivity of digydrofolate reductase from *Pneumocystis carinii* to antimicrobial agents. Abstracts of the Annual Meeting of the American Society for Microbiology, Washington, D. C., page 15.

Reinhardt, D. J., Kaplan, W., and Chandler, F. W. (1977). Morphologic resemblance of zygomycete spores to *Pneumocystis carinii* cysts in tissue. *Am. Rev. Resp. Dis.* **115**:170-172.

Rosen, P. P., Martini, N., and Armstrong, D. (1975). *Pneumocystis carinii* pneumonia. *Am. J. Med.* **58**:794-802.

Schmid, K. (1955). Zür atiologie der interstitiellen plasmocellularen pneumonie (Saccharomykose) im Sauglenepolter. *Frankf. Z. Pathol.* **66**: 426-448.

Semba, M. (1983). A reliable stain for *Pneumocystis carinii* and reticulum fibers in histologic sections. *Acta Histochem. Cytochem.* **16**:169.

Simon, H. (1953). Die Naturwissenchaften Die sagenannte *Pneumocystis carinii* eine besondere vegetationsform des Soor. *Naturwissenschaften* **40**:625-626.

Simon, H. (1955). Experimentelle untersuchungen zer frog der atiologie und pathogenese der interstitiellen plasma-cellularen pneumonie der Fruhgeburten und Sauglinge. *Verh. Dtsch. Ges. Pathol.* **38**:219.

Smith, J. W., Eichholtz, R., Miller, J., and Bartlett, M. S. (1983). Culture method for determining in vitro susceptibility of rat *Pneumocystis carinii* to pentamidine isethionate and trimethoprim sulfamethoxazole. Abstracts of the Annual Meeting of the American Society for Microbiology, New Orleans, Louisiana. American Society for Microbiology, Washington, D. C., page 21.

Sowar, M. C., and Walzer, P. D. (1982). In vitro growth studies of *Pneumocystis carinii.* Abstracts of the Interscience Conference on Antimicrobial Agents and Chemotherapy, Miami Beach, Florida. American Society for Microbiology, Washington, D.C., page 69.

Stapka, E., Wunderlich, C., and Carlson, S. (1957). Z. Morphologische and Kulturelle untersuchungen an pneumoncysten in sputum und lugenmaterial. *Z. Kinderheilkd* **79**:246-263.

Young, R. C., Bennett, J. E., and Chu, E. W. (1976). Organisms mimicking *Pneumocystis carinii. Lancet* **2**:1082-1083.

6

Clinical Aspects of Pneumocystosis in Man: Epidemiology, Clinical Manifestations, Diagnostic Approaches, and Sequelae

LOWELL S. YOUNG

University of California at Los Angeles
Center for the Health Sciences
Los Angeles, California

I. General Epidemiologic Aspects

Present concepts about the epidemiology and transmission of pneumocystis infection have been inferred from careful studies of experimentally infected animals (See Chap. 2) and clinical/serologic investigations in man. Studies demonstrating transmission of disease in animals have usually used subjects with impaired cell-mediated immunity, for example, cortisone-treated or athymic animals. These investigators support the hypothesis that infection can be transmitted by direct contact or via the airborne route (Hendley and Weller, 1971; Hughes, 1982; Walzer et al., 1977).

Most of the human epidemiologic studies have focused on clusters of cases within hospitals, orphanages, or those seen in special clinics. National surveillance data in the United States have been collected by the Centers for Disease Control, often in conjunction with the emergency distribution of pentamidine (Western et al., 1970). Some adults and children without evidence of immune deficiency have proven to have pneumocystis infection. With regard to the latter group there is mounting evidence from serologic studies that some cases of childhood pneumonia may be due to pneumocystis infection in immunocompetent patients. In one series 18% of children between 1-3 months of age, hospitalized for pneumonia appeared to have pneumocystosis (Stagno et al., 1981). While the concept that these patients were all immunologically competent has been challenged, most of them were "normal" on follow-up. An interesting cluster of infection was reported by Watanabe et al. (1965) of a family of three, two of whom died and one of whom recovered. The first case was an apparently normal 22-year-old white woman who developed fatal pneumonitis due to histologically confirmed *Pneumocystis.* Her husband developed a fatal pneumocystis infection several days later, but he had a well-documented acute lymphatic leukemia. Of interest is the 7-year-old daughter of this couple who had respiratory symptoms with diffuse lung infiltrates some two months before the onset of the infection in her parents. It has been speculated that the child was actually the index case and may have transmitted disease to her nonimmune parents, one of whom was compromised by a fatal hematologic malignancy.

With the exception of the above cluster, much of the human evidence favoring a contagious process derives from well-recorded studies of epidemic disease occurring in nurseries and orphanages in central Europe and Iran during and after the World War II (Dutz, 1970; Gajdusek, 1957). In such instances, the common denominators appear to have been overcrowding, protein calorie malnutrition, and prematurity.

In the United States, there have been three well-studied institutional outbreaks that have occurred in cancer treatment centers. The term "outbreak" is used advisably because it cannot be concluded with certainty that cases were related. The largest experience has been at the St. Jude's Childrens' Research Hospital, where large numbers of pneumocystis infection have been documented over a period of years. Epidemiologic investigations failed to establish a basis for spread of infection, but the most logical conclusion was that cases of disease arose from reactivation of latent infection triggered by the nature of the anticancer treatment (Perera et al., 1970). It is not known why some institutions that use antileukemia treatment protocols identical to those developed at St. Jude's have experienced a low incidence of documented pneumocystis infections. A somewhat different conclusion was reached with a smaller number of cases studied by Singer et al. (1975), who noted 11 histologically documented cases over a three-month interval at the Memorial Sloan-Kettering Cancer Center. Investigators of this cluster included serologic studies of patients and hospital personnel. Evidence of high antibody titers, by the indirect immunofluorescence (IFA) technique, was found in one physician and "some" nursing personnel, suggesting inapparent infection in normal subjects who could still serve as the source of infection for immunocompromised subjects. A similar outbreak occurred in a hospital treating childhood leukemia patients. Ten cases over a two-month period were investigated with serologic techniques and inapparent infections or a carrier state were suggested by high titers in medical and nursing personnel (Ruebush et al., 1978).

In our own experience, we studied several family contacts with patients who developed histologically confirmed pneumocystis infection either inside or outside of the hospital. Most family contacts did not have elevated titers (normal range in our study was an IFA titer of 1:16). We did observe one leukemic patient and three close family contacts who had high titers ($\geqslant$1:64) of immunofluorescent antibodies against a human pneumocyst antigen; none of the family members were symptomatic.

From the serologic studies of Meuwissen et al. (1977) and Stagno and collaborators (1981), it seems likely that pneumocystis infection is a common occurrence among young children. As Meuwissen has reported, close to 100% of subjects had antibody against a human cyst antigen by age 4 years. Thus, it has been inferred that in normal subjects, *Pneumocystis* is a common infection but is well handled in individuals who have intact host defense mechanisms. Institutional outbreaks, such as those occurring in orphanages, could be a manifestation of person-to-person or airborne transmission among immunologically naive subjects.

The "classic" outbreaks in institutionalized premature infants occurred in subjects experiencing onset of symptoms between the 2nd to 6th month of age, with a peak onset in the 3rd and 4th months. Of the initial 16 cases reported by Vanek and Jirovec (all of these were histopathologically confirmed), 12 were acquired in the hospital and were apparently nosocomial and 4 infections were community acquired (Vanek and Jirovec, 1952). Because of the insidious episode of infections in this group of patients, estimates of the time interval between presumed exposure and onset of symptoms vary between 20 and 80 days (Gajdusek, 1957).

In addition to the airborne (Hughes, 1982) or interpersonal spread, it has been suggested that the agent passes to the newborn from a clinically inapparent infection of the genital tract of the mother or via mother's milk, but efforts to isolate or identify the cyst/trophozoite forms in such secretions have not been successful or reproducible (Gajdusek, 1957).

Although the epidemic form of pneumocystis infection has classically been associated with the post-World War II period, it should be remembered that conditions of infant overcrowding and malnutrition persist today. Of 39 South African children who died with kwashiorkor, three or 7.7% were found to be harboring *P. carinii,* whereas no organisms were found in the lungs of 21 well-nourished and geographically matched children (Hughes et al., 1974). Equally interesting has been the documentation of pneumocystis infections in young Vietnamese infants airlifted to the United States in the Spring of 1975. Two such children, both aged 3 months, were reported by Giebink and associates (1976), and an investigation by the U.S. Centers for

Disease Control had revealed 7 verified cases of pneumocystis pneumonia in this group of refugees (Centers for Disease Control, 1976). The published studies of these patients did not identify a clear-cut immunologic disorder, but, as expected, the infants studied by Giebink were malnourished and had recent histories of diarrhea and serious bacterial infection.

In contrast to the institutional outbreaks in young premature infants the logical explanation for the large number of cases seen in immunosuppressed patients and occasional case clusters is reactivation of latent infection. Reactivation of latent infection might occur in a group of subjects with similar underlying disease managed with the same immunosuppressive drug protocol, on a specialty ward of a hospital, for example, the acute leukemia treatment unit. This might produce the appearance of "outbreak" when no spread has actually occurred. Carriers of disease must exist to explain the acquisition of antibody in healthy children, and carriers could be healthy nursing or medical personnel who demonstrate no evidence of symptomatic infection. They might in fact, acquire such inapparent infections as a result of their work if they were previously seronegative. In sporadic instances, institutional outbreaks or person-to-person spread may follow reactivation of infection in a so-called index case. It does seem clear, however, that cases of pneumocystosis have still occurred in patients managed in "protected environments" with laminar air flow, thereby giving support to the "reactivation" hypothesis.

II. Epidemiologic Data on Incidence and Underlying Disease: CDC Data

Most reports on the epidemiology of human pneumocystis infections, particularly in association with underlying diseases, emanate from major centers for the treatment of patients with neoplastic diseases, or from data gathered coincidental with the distribution of pentamidine by the U.S. Centers for Disease Control. In these cases, the information is derived almost exclusively from biopsy- or autopsy-confirmed cases. It must be recognized that such cources of information could introduce a factor of bias, because inclusion of patients in whom appropriate diagnostic procedures were attempted are often those being managed in these "tertiary care" medical referral centers. Thus, epidemiologic information and data on clinical manifestations should be regarded as relating primarily to those in whom invasive diagnostic approaches have been carried out. Admittedly, a significant population of individuals with mild disease and/or who were treated empirically with agents such as trimethoprim-sulfamethoxazole would, by definition, be excluded from analysis.

Based on observations from the Centers for Disease Control it appears that the attack rate of *Pneumocystis* is highest in the age group less than 1 year old. Most of these young patients have a primary immunodeficiency (e.g., Bruton's hypogammaglobulinemia), and following the age of 1 year the attack rate declines. Overall, leukemia was the most common underlying disease and was present in 91 of 194 cases surveyed by the CDC (Walzer et al., 1976). Hodgkin's disease and other lymphomas constituted the second most common group of underlying diseases and they are followed in third place by primary immunological deficiencies. The recipients of organ transplants were the fourth largest group of patients. The attack rate for patients with acute leukemias were as follows: 1.1% per year for acute lymphatic disease; 0.5% per year for chronic lymphatic disease; and 0.2% per year for acute myelocytic leukemia. These data are consistent with the widespread clinical impression that the disease is far more common in patients with impaired T-lymphocyte function than those with defective granulocyte bactericidal function. Our own experience has been that the occurrence of histologically proven pneumocystis infection in a patient with acute myelocytic leukemia is an extremely rare event unless the patient has received antecedent or concomitant corticosteroid therapy. Since corticosteroids now appear to be used less commonly to treat acute myelocytic leukemia, this observation could be useful in clinical decision making. Further, it should be noted that patients with acute lymphatic leukemias have a generally better prognosis than patients with acute myelocytic disease. Since they may have considerable longer survival than patients with myelocytic leukemia, they are at even greater risk for contracting pneumocystis infection. Interestingly, the risk of pneumocystis infection does not necessarily relate to control of underlying disease. As has been pointed out by Hughes and collaborators, prior to the introduction of effective chemoprophylaxis, pneumocystis pneumonia was the most common documented microbial cause of infection in patients with childhood lymphatic leukemia in the remission state (Hughes et al., 1973). Additionally, the risk of *Pneumocystis* could have been compounded by the use of corticosteroids in high dose, which is still conventional therapy given to patients in remission. Other childhood diseases for which corticosteroids are commonly administered (e.g., nephrotic syndrome), do not seem to be as closely associated with risk of pneumocystis infection, although a comparative study of incidence between that syndrome and acute leukemia has not been carried out.

One important area of interest relates to whether or not cellular or humoral deficiencies or both seem to predispose to pneumocystis infection. Clearly some impairment to both limbs of the immune system can be found in many patients with pneumocystis infection, but Burke and Good, commenting on their extensive experience with *Pneumocystis* (46 childhood and adult cases at one medical center), express the view that the defect "most commonly associated with pneumocystis infection of the sporadic type is a deficiency of humoral immune mechanisms" (Burke and Good, 1973). They noted that by 1973 only one case of pneumocystis infection with a pure T-cell deficiency, thymic aplasia, had been reported and that *Pneumocystis* is an extreme rarity in pure thymic aplasia as manifested in the DiGeorge syndrome. They noted also that in the reported cases of pneumocystis pneumonia reviewed by 1973, 53 had hypogammaglobulinemia only, while only 13 had severe combined immunodeficiency, and 1 had absent cell-mediated immunity. On the other hand, Schultz (1976), commenting upon the CDC data reported by Walzer and colleagues (1973) found that quite to the contrary from an epidemiologic analysis of cases treated with pentamidine in the United States, there was no apparent difference in incidence between disorders of humoral and antibody synthesis versus those with impaired mononuclear cell or delayed hypersensitivity defense mechanisms. Most likely then, differences in association between immunodeficiency states and pneumocystis infection could represent institutional differences and patterns of hospital referral as well as local epidemiologic factors.

III. Epidemiologic Aspects of an Outbreak of *Pneumocystis carinii* Pneumonia in Patients with Apparent Acquired Immunodeficiency

There have been few exceptions to the observation that pneumocystis pneumonia occurs almost exclusively in patients with a well-defined immunodeficient state. For instance, Walzer and colleagues reviewed requests to the U.S. Centers for Disease Control for pentamidine in the period 1967-1970 when it was the only recommended treatment for Pneumocystis pneumonia. They found only a single case of documented infection in a patient without an established underlying disease (Walzer et al., 1976). Additionally, some patients have come to medical attention with diffuse pneumonia which eventually proved to be due to *Pneumocystis*. It is only at this or some subsequent date that the individual is found to have an underlying neoplasm such as a lymphoma.

One of the most dramatic increases of pneumocystis infections in patients without previously established underlying disease has recently been documented in a number of hospitals. Since June 1981, the U.S. Centers for Disease Control have collected data on an increasing number of cases of *Pneumocystis carinii* pneumonia, often in association with Kaposi's sarcoma and other serious opportunistic infections. An elaborate, but still imprecise surveillance program has identified a total of 91 cases of pneumocystis pneumonia, and almost an identical number (98) of Kaposi's sarcoma and 18 patients who had both conditions (Centers for Disease Control, 1982). The numbers of cases appear to be increasing rapidly. The mortality rate in these patients has exceeded 40%, but it is not clear whether deaths have been attributed solely to pneumocystis infection or the underlying neoplastic disease. Of the important epidemiologic observations thus far, perhaps the most striking is that the great majority of cases have occurred in cities in California and New York but few cases have been documented in a number of tertiary care centers in other areas of the United States. In the four-year period 1976-1980, there was but one request to the CDC for pentamidine to treat an adult without an underlying disease, but in 1981 alone there were 42 such requests. These represented more than a third of all of the requests for pentamidine in the United States. Of interest is that recurrent *Pneumocystis carinii* pneumonia was documented in 8 patients, of whom 4 died. In those cases with both Kaposi's sarcoma and pneumocystis pneumonia one or the other process antedated the other by several months. Almost all of the reported cases have occurred in men, and more than 90% of these subjects reported to be homosexual or bisexual when sexual preference could be elicited. Most of these individuals were previously in good health, hence the supposition that the factors predisposing to *Pneumocystis* were "acquired."

A remarkable observation in association with this outbreak has been the presence of other serious opportunistic infections. These apparent copathogens are microbes against which cell-mediated immune functions has been thought to be critical in host defense. These include herpes simplex virus, *Toxoplasma gondii*, *Cryptococcus neoformans*, *Candida albicans*, mycobacteria of several "atypical" types, cryptosporidia, and cytomegalovirus (CMV). The single largest group of concurrent infectious processes was cytomegalovirus infection confirmed by virus isolation or biopsy. A greater number of individuals have had high serum antibody titers or demonstrated seroconversion against the virus antigen, suggesting an even higher incidence of this infectious process.

The simultaneous occurrence of Kaposi's sarcoma and pneumocystis pneumonia among homosexual men in the same age and racial groups who live in the same geographical areas has strongly suggested the occurrence of a single epidemic of underlying immunosuppression. The first detailed clinical reports about this outbreak were simultaneously published at the end of 1981 and include the report of Masur and associates describing 11 cases in men without previous underlying disorders or therapy. Although 6 of these men were homosexuals, 5 others were reported to be drug abusers (Masur et al., 1981). Gottlieb and colleagues studied a similar population and found cutaneous anergy to a number of skin test antigens, decreased responses upon in vitro stimulation of lymphocytes to phytohemagglutin and concanavalin A, and decreased ratios of helper to suppressor T lymphocytes in four patients with pneumocystis pneumonia (Gottlieb et al., 1981). Similar evidence of depressed cellular immunity was reported by Siegel and collaborators (1981) using other techniques in 15 additional patients.

Thus, reports of a dramatic increase in pneumocystis infection in individuals without previously documented underlying disease or depressed host defense mechanisms have represented the most important development in the epidemiology of this disease during the past decade. Unfortunately, information on the immunologic status of such patients prior to the documentation of either pneumocystis pneumonia or Kaposi's sarcoma is not available. There has been intense speculation as to the mechanism for the apparently acquired immunodeficiency. While much attention has focused on either intravenous or inhalation drug abuse, it has been well demonstrated that the cytomegalovirus induces transient abnormalities in cellular immune function in otherwise healthy individuals and that evidence of CMV infection or shedding of this virus has been quite common in homosexual men (Drew et al., 1981). Clearly, other studies have demonstrated an increased susceptibility to infection following CMV infection in experimental model systems (Bale et al., 1982; Hamilton et al., 1976). While a plausible hypothesis is that CMV infection precedes or predisposes to reactivation of latent pneumocystis infection, this hypothesis still needs to be tested in prospective epidemiologic studies. In patients who have received organ transplants, it has been well appreciated that CMV and pneumocystis infection can occur simultaneously or be closely associated (Rand et al., 1978). Additionally, cytomegalovirus infection is quite common among adults in the United States and increasing prevalence of seropositivity with age has been demonstrated. Whether a particular strain of the virus or the virus acting in concordance with an unusual type of drug abuse may predispose to pneumocystis infection, some of the other infections, and neoplastic phenomena, remains a subject of intense concern. Even if such were demonstrated, the underlying mechanisms behind the sudden temporal appearance of these infections in a predominantly homosexual population remain to be elucidated. (See Chapter 8.)

With renewed worldwide interest in pneumocystis infection, increased efforts at finding cases of infections in individuals with "acquired immunodeficiency" now cast doubt on the exclusive association of this new syndrome with homosexuality. Few cases have occurred in homosexual females and documented pneumocystosis in heterosexual males and females with evidence of acquired immunodeficiency have also occurred. Whether this most recent phenomena represents a "spillover" of an epidemic of acquired immunosuppression to the nonhomosexual population has been widely speculated. The most recent occurrence of pneumocystis infection in multiply transfused patients with hemophilia A (but no history of drug abuse or homosexuality) is both striking and ominous (Centers for Disease Control, 1982). It suggests that there may be an agent transmitted by blood transfusions that predisposes toward acquired immunosuppression and reactivation of latent infection, or that *Pneumocystis* itself could spread by the transfusion route.

IV. Clinical Manifestations of Pneumocystis Infection

Irrespective of underlying disease, there are no distinctive clinical features which identify *Pneumocystis carinii* as the etiologic agent of pulmonary infection. The signs and symptoms of extensive pulmonary involvement are quite variable in different hosts and it is likely that the degree of therapeutic immunosuppression given to some patients tends to mask the presence of far advanced, sometimes fatal pneumocystis infection. The finding that pneumocystis infection complicates an immunosuppressed state makes it likely that there will often be concurrent infectious processes. However, associated processes need not be infectious in etiology. Besides tumor, radiation pneumonitis and drug reactions can mimic pneumocystosis. The widespread use of chemotherapeutic agents such as bleomycin in patients with lymphoid neoplasms may result in a diffuse pneumonitis which represents a reaction to that drug. Such patients have often received lung radiation. The clinical picture is indistinguishable from clinical pneumocystis infection. It is not unusual to see *Pneumocystis* developing in a lympnoma patient who has had prior radiation and bleomycin therapy. All three processes—drug reaction, radiation pneumonitis, and pneumocystis infection may be present in the same patient.

The classic "epidemic" type of infection in orphans cared for in foundling homes was reported to be rather slow and insidious in onset. Initial signs were nonspecific, such as restlessness, lethargy, and poor feeding. The reports of Dutz and collaborators documented the evolution of this clinical syndrome over a period of weeks, evolving into significant symptomatology with tachypnea, severe dyspnea, periorbital and perioral cyanosis (Dutz et al., 1976). It was noted that cough was highly variable and fever was initially absent or low grade. Within one to two weeks a more florid clinical picture developed, characterized by dyspnea, nasal alae fold dilitation, sternal retraction, use of accessory muscles for breathing, and marked tachypnea. Cyanosis became more pronounced and a more exhausting nonproductive cough occurred in spasms and became a regular feature. One of the more striking clinical observations in the orphanage studies was an apparent difference between respiratory symptoms and auscultatory findings, with a minimum of auscultatory findings despite significant dyspnea and progressive lung infiltrates involving most of the areas of the lung. In these studies the total duration of symptomatology prior to diagnosis and initiation of treatment often exceeded a month.

A "typical" clinical syndrome has not been readily identifiable in the usual sporadic cases of pneumocystis infection occurring in both children and adults throughout the United States. In the series reported by Burke and Good from the University of Minnesota Hospitals, both a slow and insidious onset of infection (corresponding to the cases occurring in orphanages) and an abrupt, fulminating type of illness were reported (Burke and Good, 1973). Some children with underlying congenital immunodeficiency diseases appeared to have insidious onset of symptoms similar to the epidemic form of infection, and some of these cases had protracted symptoms several months prior to diagnosis. By contrast, children and most adults with severe underlying diseases, such as neoplasms and acquired defects in host defenses, often experienced an abrupt onset of illness with high fevers, tachypnea, and cough which progressed to a fatal outcome even with treatment. Immunosuppression, however, did not always lead to more severe onset of disease and the use of corticosteroids may have suppressed the initial clinical manifestations of infection. Our own experience with corticosteroid therapy as well as the experience of others suggests that a "flare" in respiratory symptoms heralding the onset of pneumocystis infection can follow a reduction or discontinuation of steroid dosage. The most plausible explanation for this often repeated observation is that steroids exert an anti-inflammatory effect. While clearly predisposing to pneumocystosis the manifestations of infection are retarded until steroid dose is reduced, a phenomena which may be conceived as "desuppression."

The signs and symptoms of pneumocystis pneumonia have been summarized in Table 1 (Walzer et al., 1976). This information is based on the survey of the Centers for Disease Control of case report forms of patients treated with pentamidine. The most common symptom of pneumocystis pneumonia was dyspnea which was present in 91% of the patients. Fever was present, however, in only two-thirds of the patients and cough was present in one-half. Perhaps more interesting, only 7% of the patients had productive cough and only 2 patients in this series had hemoptysis. In a great majority of children, tachypnea with a respiratory rate exceeding 40 per minute was present as well as a weak dry cough. Similar to the epidemic form of disease, the absence of characteristic rales was occasionally observed in spite of extensive pulmonary involvement documented radiologically. Overall, rales were detected in only 33% of patients. Another finding in the CDC summary deserves comment: the hepatomegaly noted in a third and splenomegaly in a fifth of the patients were most likely due to under-

Table 1 Signs, Symptoms, and Radiologic Features of 168 Patients with Histologically Confirmed Pneumocystis Pneumonia (Center for Disease Control Summary)

Clinical features	Number of patients	Percent
Symptoms		
Dyspnea	152	91
Fever	110	66
Cough	79	47
Productive cough	12	7
Hemoptysis	3	2
Chest pain	11	7
Night sweats	1	1
Signs (respiratory)		
Cyanosis	66	39
Rales	56	33
Breath sounds		
Decreased	22	13
Bronchial/tubular	14	8
Dullness	9	5
Ronchi	7	4
Wheezing	2	1
Signs (other)		
Hepatomegaly	59	35
Splenomegaly	32	19
X-ray		
Infiltrate		
Diffuse and bilateral	164	98
Unilateral	4	2
Effusion	8	5
Adventitious air[a]	6	4

[a]Pneumothorax, pneumomediastinum, etc.
Source: Walzer et al. (1976).

lying disease, such as a neoplastic process. Additionally, Hughes and collaborators have noted a high incidence of mediastinal lymphadenopathy in their patients which could be due to concurrent neoplastic involvement (Hughes et al., 1975). Their data emphasizes, however, that the presence of hilar adenopathy on chest x-ray does not exclude the concurrent presence of pneumocystis infection in the lung parenchyma. One finding observed by Hughes and colleagues at St. Jude's Research Hospital, primarily a center for the therapy of neoplastic disorders in children, was that 21% of their patients had mild diarrhea at the onset or during the course of pneumocystis pneumonitis (Hughes et al., 1973). Possibly, some of these symptoms may have been due to other medications that were given, such as antimicrobial agents.

One of the most prevalent beliefs, particularly among physicians caring for individuals receiving immunosuppressive or antineoplastic therapy, is that pneumocystis infection is a fulminant process. Nonetheless, in the CDC analysis, the duration of symptoms in 153 patients with confirmed pneumocystis infection ranged from less than 7 to greater than 90 days with a median of approximately 13 days (Walzer et al., 1976). Thus, if one carefully searches out symptoms, a considerable number of patients will give considerably premonitory signals of the clinical "flare" in their disease. The onset of symptoms such as mild nonproductive cough and/or dyspnea should be viewed with suspicion even though patients may not be febrile. In our experience, we have observed several patients who made repeated visits to a hospital emergency room because of spells of coughing, tachypnea, or dyspnea. Chest roentgenograms were initially negative or revealed only minor abnormalities. The cursory management of such patients without x-ray findings in the emergency rooms cannot really be faulted, but such signs and symptoms were actually the first warnings of incipient pneumocystis infection. Clearly, such examples indicate that frank pulmonary infiltrates can "lag behind" the infection of the lung parenchyma. Reports to the effect that gallium scans of the lung have been abnormal prior to the development of infiltrates further support the concept of such a sequence of events. In fact, lung biopsies carried out for abnormal gallium scans of the lungs but without a clear pulmonary infiltrate have led to early diagnosis of pneumocystis infection (Levenson et al., 1976; Turbiner et al., 1978; Fossieck and Spangnslo, 1980).

Hughes and collaborators (1975) have well documented the risk of pneumocystis pneumonia in relation to the type of antileukemic therapy given for various stages in the treatment of the disease. At a time when acute lymphatic leukemia was treated only with steroids, vincristine, and L-asparginase, no patient out of a total of 149 receiving that particular protocol developed pneumocystosis. When the protocol was changed to include additional intrathecal methotrexate and central nervous system irradiation, this group experienced 4% incidence of pneumocystis infection. Consolidation therapy over an ensuing 2-3-year period involved randomization to four treatment groups. A 5% incidence of pneumocystosis was noted when the maintenance therapy consisted of methotrexate with or without 6-mercapto-purine and cyclophosphamide. However, when cytosine arabinoside was added to methotrexate, 6-mercaptopurine, and cyclophosphamide, 22.4% of 41 children developed histologically documented pneumocystis pneumonia. The obvious conclusion is that the incidence of pneumocystis infection in leukemic children reflected the intensity of immunosuppression. While it might be assumed that this would be true for all infectious complications in this high-risk group of patients, it was not borne out by their experience. Hughes and colleagues have contrasted the incidence of varicella-zoster infection and pneumocystis pneumonia in leukemic children (Hughes et al., 1975). Whereas the latter described group of intensely treated leukemic children had almost a 25% incidence of pneumocystis infection, they experienced no increased risk of varicella-zoster infection.

With regard to underlying disease and nature of immunosuppression, it appears that increasing numbers of patients who traditionally have not been thought to be prone to pneumocystis infection have developed histologically documented disease. This is most likely due to the extension of immuno-suppressive therapy to treat diseases where previously this type of approach was uncommon. We have observed cases in patients with severe inflammatory dermatologic disorders treated with high doses of corticosteroids and cyto-toxic agents. Among patients with neoplastic diseases there are reports of histologically confirmed infections in individuals with neoplasms such as bronchogenic carcinoma (Fossieck and Spangnslo, 1980). Review of the treatment protocols in the 5 cases reveals a common theme that all patients had been treated with combination antineoplastic therapy, but in 2, treatment did not include corticosteroids. This emphasizes that while corticosteroids appear to be an important predisposing factor in most of the reported cases, pneumocystis infection can occur in malignant processes without steroids being given.

V. Laboratory Findings

Despite the ever-increasing number of laboratory tests available in modern hospitals, there are no abnormalities that point toward the likelihood of pneumocystis infection. Patients are often anemic, leukopenic, or thrombocytopenic, but these abnormalities result from an underlying disease or its treatment. In some patients with primary immune deficiency disease it has been claimed that pneumocystis infection may trigger significant eosinophilia (Burke and Good, 1975). However, this finding is not typical of patients with underlying malignancies. Eosinophilia may be a manifestation of other infectious processes (e.g., toxoplasmosis, strongyloides, coccidioidomycosis) or of neoplasms such as Hodgkin's disease. A few cases of pneumocystis infection have been associated with hypercalcemia, but this has not turned out to be a reliable diagnostic clue. Clearly, hypercalcemia may be a reflection of bone involvement with neoplasm. Additionally, elevated cold agglutinin titers have been noted in some cases of epidemic disease or in recipients of renal transplants who developed *Pneumocystis*. It is apparently not a common finding, and cold agglutinins may become detectable following mycoplasma or many viral infections.

Pathophysiologic changes accompanying pneumocystis infection are similar to those reported in other diffuse pulmonary infections. Disorders of ventilation and perfusion are compatible with the so-called "alveolar-capillary block syndrome." Arterial blood gas determination usually shows severe hypoxemia and hypercapnia. Terminally, respiratory acidosis is commonly observed.

Lyons and colleagues performed a complete battery of pulmonary function tests in one case of pneumocystis pneumonia whom they reported had no predisposing underlying disease (Lyons et al., 1961). Their findings included a low lung compliance combined with normal nonelastic resistance. This indicated a "rigid lung" without elements of obstruction. These abnormalities were felt to be similar to that observed in the Hamman-Rich syndrome. Another recent review published by Doak et al. (1973) involved detailed pulmonary function tests in recipients of cadaveric renal allografts who developed what was called "transplant lung." Actually, *Pneumocystis* was found to be responsible for the majority of these episodes of posttransplantation pneumonitis. Besides hypoxemia an increased alveolar to arterial oxygen tension difference was a consistent finding. Frank ventilatory failure, as measured by CO_2 accumulation did not occur until the terminal stages of infection. It appeared that hypoxia resulted from gross hypoventilation of perfused lungs. Both reduced diffusing capacity and decreased compliance were also demonstrable in a few patients.

As has been emphasized in many reviews and a prior segment of this chapter, pneumocystis infection may present concurrently with other infectious processes. Half of the patients with pneumocystis infection also had a concurrent infection in a series reported by the Centers for Disease Control (Walzer et al., 1976). Cytomegalovirus infection (CMV) appears to be the most common process associated with pneumocystosis. This was first identified by Gajdusek in his initial review published in 1957 and has been reconfirmed in many studies including the recent cases of pneumocystosis associated with acquired immunodeficiency (Centers for Disease Control, 1982). Table 2, while summarizing some of the infections which must be considered

Table 2 Differential Diagnosis of Diffuse Pulmonary Infiltrates in the Compromised Host

Bacterial
    Aerobic and anaerobic cocci
    Gram-negative bacilli
    Mycobacteria
    Nocardial asteroides
    Legionella pneumophila

Fungi
    Aspergillus fumigatus
    Zygomycetes
    Petriellidium boydii
    Candida sp.
    Cryptococcus neoformans
    Histoplasma capsulatum
    Coccidioides immitis

Parasites
    Pneumocystis carinii
    Toxoplasma gondii
    Strongyloides stercoralis

Viruses
    Cytomegalovirus
    Herpes simplex
    Varicella zoster
    Adenovirus
    Rubeola

Other Processes
    Pulmonary edema
    Leukoagglutinin reactions
    Drug toxicity: bleomycin, busulfan, nitrofurantoin
    Radiation fibrosis
    Oxygen toxicity
    Neoplasm
    Hemorrhage

in the differential diagnosis of diffuse pulmonary infiltrates, is also a list of concurrent infectious processes that can occur in patients with pneumocystosis. The DNA viruses, particularly CMV, varicella-zoster and herpes simplex are common. Gram-negative and gram-positive pneumonias, fungal pneumonias, and other protozoal infections such as toxoplasmosis may occur simultaneously.

VI. Diagnosis of Pneumocystis Infection

At the time that the diagnosis of pneumocystis infection is considered the patient is often seriously or critically ill. An underlying disease is usually present which may be poorly controlled but occasionally may be in remission (as often occurs with acute lymphocytic leukemia of childhood). It goes without saying that every clinician who deals with these situations would like to have a safe, inexpensive, easily obtainable, highly accurate diagnostic procedure to confirm the presence of the pneumocystis infection. While a "dipstick" test to diagnose pneumocystis infection would be a great boon to clinical management, none is available nor is it likely that one will be developed. Pneumocystis pneumonia is one of the most difficult respiratory infections to diagnose and usually requires an invasive procedure to obtain pulmonary secretions of direct samples of lung parenchyma. Other sections of this book (Chap. 4) are devoted to the serologic diagnosis of pneumocystis infection utilizing both antigen detection and antibody response recognition methods. Antigen detection systems clearly need further work, whereas measurements of antibody are insensitive in a significant portion of immunodeficient patients with proven disease. While serial antibody measurements might be valuable in "recouping" the diagnosis in patients too ill to undergo diagnostic procedures who were empirically treated, they are probably of limited value in acute clinical disease and are available only through certain referral centers.

One of the paradoxes in the management of the patient with diffuse pulmonary infiltrates is that while the lung is one of the "most visible" of the deep organs, pulmonary tissues are relatively inaccessible and specific diagnosis of intrapulmonary pathology requires an invasive procedure. Compounding this problem is that multiple pathological and infectious processes may be present simultaneously in an immunocompromised host. Successful diagnosis of one of these processes (e.g., recovery of nocardial organisms from subcutaneous abscess in a patient who also has pneumonia) or the measurement of an elevated antibody titers against *Histoplasma capsulatum* or cytomegalovirus may be of limited value in diagnosing accurately a lung infiltrate—which by itself may be caused by several organisms. The detection

Table 3 Open Lung Biopsy for Diffuse Infiltrates

Etiology	Study by year of publication			
	NCI,[a] 1970 (Goodell et al., 1970)	Sloan-Kettering, 1975 (Rosen et al., 1975)	NCI,[b] 1978 (Leight and Michaelis, 1978)	Wisconsin, 1981 (Jaffe and Maki, 1981)
Pneumocystis carinii	8	18	10	6 (8[a])
Aspergillus sp.	1	2	2	1
Aspergillus/CMV	2			
Cytomegalovirus (CMV)	2		3	4[b]
Bacterial pneumonia	1	3	3	4
Cryptococcus	1	1		
Candida sp.		2	2	
Rubeola	1			
Toxoplasma gondii	1			
Neoplasm	1	5	3	4
Allergic reaction, edema bronchiolitis		3		
Mycobacteria			1	
Toxic pneumonitis			3	2
Other identified causes	1		3	2
Cause unknown	3	15	12	3

[a]National Cancer Institute.
[b]2 patients had both pneumocystis and CMV.

of one infectious process and its successful treatment surely does not exclude the presence of other concomitant infecting or supervening processes. One major clinical mistake often repeated is to assume that after a patient demonstrates a clinical response to treatment of a documented infection, the return of pulmonary signs and fever is due to relapse of that initially diagnosed process rather than a new one.

Differential diagnosis of the cause of the diffuse pulmonary infiltrates includes a number of infectious and noninfectious entities that are shown in Table 2. Large series of reports on pneumocystis infection or in studies of diffuse lung infiltrates identify *Pneumocystis* as one of the leading causes of such diffuse infiltrates and are summarized in Table 3. It is true that some of the entities listed in these tables can be diagnosed by noninvasive serologic techniques, and it goes without saying that rapid attempts to exclude these other agents are clearly indicated in the early stages of the evaluation of the patients with diffuse pneumonitis.

VII. Initial Diagnostic Approaches

The classic approach for evaluating the patient with pneumonia includes a history, physical examination, an examination and culture of sputum, and roentgenologic studies. There are major limitations to each of these approaches that have become all too apparent in the management of the compromised host. This history may be of some value if a patient has had contact with other individuals with a documented respiratory infection, if there have been outbreaks of respiratory infection in the community, or an extended circule of contacts. For diagnosis of *Pneumocystis,* a history of drug treatment for an underlying disease is important. In the case of recipients of steroids, recent dosage reductions can occasionally be a valuable clue since "tapering" of steroids has been associated with "flaring" of clinical disease. Physical examination can establish the presence of pulmonary disease, but unfortunately provides few clues to etiology of infection. In addition to regular chest films, radioisotopic scanning of lung with gallium may define the presence of diffuse pulmonary abnormalities even before lung infiltrates are detectable (Turbiner et al., 1978; Fossieck and Spangnslo, 1980). This could be of some value in the hypoxic patient with a clear chest x-ray in differentiating pneumocystosis from pulmonary emboli.

Sputum examination and culture can be misleading. Even with pneumococcal pneumonia, individuals with concomitant pneumococcal bacteremia may not have gram-positive cocci in their expectorated sputum. *Pneumocystis* organisms have been infrequently detected in sputum although isolated examples do exist (Lau et al., 1976). Nonetheless, it seems prudent in the evaluation of the immunocompromised host who may have *Pneumocystis* to expend the effort to evaluate sputum if available, and to attach some significance to the bacteriologic strains if neutrophils and pulmonary alveolar macrophages are present which suggest parenchymal lung disease. On the other hand, specimens containing squamous epithelial cells represent material from the upper pharyngeal passages and the value of the examination should be seriously questioned. Fluorescent screening of sputum for presence of pneumocysts with highly specific antiserum has been proposed by Lim et al. (1974), but the antiserum and its potency and reliability are still factors which would not lead this to be a common, widely performed test.

VIII. Radiologic Manifestations of Pneumocystis Pneumonia

In most series of patients with proven pneumocystis pneumonia clearcut chest roentgenologic abnormalities have been present. Some noteworthy exceptions have been reported (see below) as well as some cases, reported by Hughes and colleagues where autopsies performed after 48 hours of normal chest x-rays revealed *P. carinii* pneumonitis (Forrest, 1972).

The typical clinical picture of pneumocystis involvement of the lung is a diffuse, bilateral, alveolar-interstitial reticulonodular pneumonitis that is progressive and coalescing. The infiltrate usually begins in the perihilar area and the initial changes may give a "ground glass" appearance. With progression of disease there is radiation of infiltrates from these central foci into both lung fields. Frequently there is apical sparing and occasionally there is a relative sparing of both the apexes and bases, with the infiltrate presenting as a truly perihilar process in a "butterfly pattern." From an initial patchy reticulogranular appearance, there is progression of disease to more diffuse, fluffy, alveolar consolidation pattern and finally to dense lobar consolidation. Many radiologic experts have commented on the inaccuracy of referring to pneumocystis pneumonia as a predominantly interstitial process (Forrest, 1972; Dee et al., 1979; Doppmann and Geelhoed, 1976). The pattern of involvement is usually a combination of alveolar or airspace consolidation with a less striking interstitial component of cellular infiltration or edema. Early involvement of the alveoli is patchy, and thus may be confused with an interstitial infiltrate on the chest film, but rapid progression leads to coalescence and appearance of air bronchograms. In more than half of the patients in one series, air bronchograms were present (Doppmann and Geelhoed, 1976). The progression to dense alveolar consolidation usually evolves over a 3-5 day period.

In the infant pneumocystis syndrome associated with prematurity and crowding, Paldy and Ivady described six distinct stages of pneumocystosis (Paldy and Ivady, 1976). They commented that these radiologic stages can be correlated only indirectly with pathologic findings and that the syndrome appeared to evolve more slowly than that observed in the frankly immuno-deficient patients now more commonly seen. "Stage I" was described as prominence of bronchial and vascular outlines slowly evolving within 3 or 4 weeks to stage II. The second stage was characterized by further bronchial-vascular enlargement, pinhead-size atelectatic spots, and an "interstitial net-work" visible in the peripheral portion of the lungs. Stage III was charac-terized by intense networklike opacity at interstices linking bronchial and vascular outlines, inflation of the peripheral parts of the lung, flattening of the dome of the diaphragm, increased lung volume, emphysema, and en-hanced lung opacity. In this stage, pinhead-size spots and larger shadows may alternate with emphysematous spots and in the PA x-ray projection a "butterfly" distribution could be observed. Stage IV was found to evolve over 3-5 days, and was characterized by hyperinflation of the lung, more pronounced diaphragmatic flattening, widening of the intercostal spaces, al-ternating areas of atelectasis, opacity of the interstitial spaces, and visible air bronchograms (a picture that could be confused with miliary tuberculosis). Stage V is described as the "crisis stage," it is achieved in several days from stage IV during which interstitial, peribronchial, and perivascular infiltrates develop in addition to various degrees of alveolar filling, atelectasis, and em-physema. Lungs are maximally distended and the coarse shadows of the in-terstitial infiltrates reach out to the periphery and basal portion of the lung. Occasionally patients may have emphysematous bullae that can rupture re-sulting in pneumothorax, mediastinitis, and cervical emphysema. Despite pneumothorax, there is no generalized lung collapse because the lungs are stiff. Thus, mediastinal shifts are uncommon. The VIth stage of Ivady and Paldy was that of slow resolution, which could take place over months fol-lowing treatment.

As pointed out by Ivady and Paldy, one of the important aspects of differential diagnosis is miliary tuberculosis, particularly in its congenital form. However, they caution that all interstitial processes of the lung may resemble pneumocystis pneumonia. The problem of nonspecificity of the lung x-ray picture is echoed in the work of Doppmann and Geelhoed (1976) who reviewed 30 cases of documented pneumocystis pneumonia and found the incidence of atypical radiologic findings to be appreciable: 17 of 30 (56%) proven cases had at least one atypical finding. For instance, 40% of patients did not show sparing of the apices, 13% had unilateral predominance of lung infiltrates, 2 had lobar segmental consolidation, 2 of 30 cases had a pseudonodular pattern, cavitation was observed in one patient (but this patient also had *Candida* present at autopsy), and two patients had hilar enlargement. They concluded that presence of large pleural effusions and cavitation were points against the diagnosis, as may be hilar adenopathy. However, the latter, hilar enlargement, was common in the experience of Hughes et al. (1975) and could reflect the underlying disease. Doppmann and Geelhoed (1976) concluded that histological confirmation is necessary in a significant portion of cases and few radiologic findings completely exclude the diagnosis of pneumocystis pneumonia. Pneumothorax is probably a more common manifestation in the childhood or infantile syndrome, but it may obviously occur along with a pneumomediastinum secondary to ventilatory support.

Table 4 summarizes some of the unusual radiologic manifestations reported in histologically proven pneumocystis infection. These unusual manifestations include cavitation, nodular lesions, lobar consolidation, pneumatoceles, interstitial emphysema, pneumothorax, and pneumomediastinum. There are some reservations about these reports, but some of them are unequivocable in their documentation of *Pneumocystis* organisms present in the histopathologic lesion. For instance, the reports of cavities have not necessarily had biopsy or autopsy material on exactly the same structure observed radiologically, or when such was possible (Rodriguez-Severa et al., 1976) other microbial pathogens were also present. As mentioned previously, the presence of pneumothorax, pneumatoceles, and pneumomediastinum may be secondary to positive pressure-assisted ventilation.

Of great interest have been those reports listed in Table 4, where apparently the pneumocystis infection was associated with a normal chest x-ray. The important clinical clues leading to diagnosis of disease in these cases were tachypnea and hypoxemia. In three of the series listed, gallium-67 lung scans were performed to evaluate incipient lung disease, metastatic neoplasia, or infection elsewhere in the body (Levenson et al., 1976; Turbiner et al., 1978; Sirotzky et al., 1978). What is remarkable in these reports is that gallium scans diagnosed lung abnormalities prior to development of a lung infiltrate. Usually the distribution of the gallium uptake was symmetrical and diffuse. Several authors (Levenson et al., 1976; Friedman et al., 1975) have commented that pneumocystis infection should be strongly suspected in an immunodeficient patient with tachypnea, hypoxemia, and a scan/radiologic discordancy. However, it should be noted that gallium patterns are hardly specific for pneumocystis infection, being positive in a wide variety of lung processes secondary to drug toxicity, pulmonary edema, and interstitial fibrosis.

Table 4 Unusual Radiologic Manifestations of Pneumocystis Infection

Finding	Reference
Asymmetric distribution	Burke and Good, 1973
Cavitation	Doppmann and Geelhoed, 1976; Siegel and Wolson, 1977
Interstitial emphysema	Luddy et al., 1977
Lobar consolidation	Burke and Good, 1973; Byrd and Horn, 1976
Nodular lesions	Cross and Steigbigel, 1974; Rodriguez-Servera et al., 1976
Normal chest x-ray	Levenson et al., 1976; Turbiner et al., 1978; Dee et al., 1979; Sirotzky et al., 1978
Pleural effusion	Burke and Good, 1973
Pneumomediastinum	Luddy et al., 1977
Pneumatocele	Luddy et al., 1977
Pneumothorax	Luddy et al., 1977

IX. The Pros and Cons of Establishing a Diagnosis of Pneumocystis Infection

Considerable controversy surrounds the indication and value of attempting a diagnostic procedure to diagnose pneumocystis infection. The principal dilemma facing the responsible physician is whether or not the high-risk patient, who is prone to develop complications such as bleeding and pneumothorax, should be subjected to an invasive procedure to establish the etiology of lung infiltrates. The alternative is to give an empiric trial of antimicrobial therapy that offers broad coverage of the likely organisms. If a decision is made to make a specific diagnosis, there is a paucity of data on the comparative accuracy and safety of various invasive procedures that have been used. Experienced clinicians recognize that failure to treat will lead to almost certain death in the high-risk patient, but choosing specific therapy involves risks of complications from an invasive diagnosis procedure that may actually accelerate the clinical deterioration of the patient.

A prudent clinical approach is one that attempts to integrate all of the clinical and laboratory information that can be rapidly marshalled, but if measures such as sputum examination and available serologic tests are uninformative then an attempt should be made to perform an invasive procedure. Until the availability of trimethoprim-sulfamethoxazole, a relatively safe agent for the initial therapy of pneumocystis infection, the argument favoring an invasive diagnostic procedure was that empiric pentamidine treatment involved considerable risk of toxicity. By excluding pneumocystis infection serious pentamidine-related complications could be avoided. Certainly there are patients whose clinical condition is so poor (severe thrombocytopenia uncorrected by platelet transfusions) that it would be unwise to attempt an invasive diagnostic procedure. It must be remembered, however, that trimethoprim-sulfamethoxazole is not specific therapy for *Pneumocystis carinii* in the sense that pentamidine was, and that clinical improvement is not of diagnostic value. This is of little practical concern to the improving patient, but an important diagnostic dilemma remains if the patient does not improve.

From several studies, summarized in Table 3, it appears that *Pneumocystis* accounts for no more than one-third of the etiologies of diffuse lung infiltrates in immunocompromised patients. Empiric therapy for pneumocystis infection when another treatable infectious or neoplastic disease is present could be disastrous. Diffuse lung infiltrates caused by mycobacteria, opportunistic fungi, and some of the viral agents are amenable to alternate chemotherapy. The recognition of new potentially treatable infections caused by agents such as *Legionella pneumophila* or *Chlamydia* species is an important reminder of the value of establishing specific diagnoses. If a patient fails to improve for reasons unrelated to the infectious process, such as oxygen toxicity, then an initial empiric course of therapy could mask an original provocative agent such as *Pneumocystis.* The insoluble dilemma is whether or not the initial presumptive diagnosis was correct, the infection has responded partially but is still the cause of lung infiltrates, or whether cysts were missed because of a sampling error of the surgical procedure that is eventually carried out. One of the real dangers is that early empirical therapy with trimethoprim-sulfamethoxazole may so confuse the clinical and histological picture, whether initially caused by *Pneumocystis* or other organisms, that the lung biopsy obtained at a later date is misleading. The studies of Sattler and Remington (1981), wherein repeat biopsies were performed in a number of patients treated with trimethoprim-sulfamethoxazole, show that cysts disappear within a few days after appropriate treatment has been started.

Some retrospective studies of the most invasive diagnostic procedure, open-lung biopsy, have failed to discern a difference in the eventual mortality in patients subjected to this procedure who had a specific diagnosis made versus those who did not, or between those whose treatment was altered because a diagnosis was established versus those in whom the results of biopsy did not effect treatment (Rossiter et al., 1979). Nonetheless, such information does not necessarily lead to a conclusion that open-lung biopsy is without value, since the patients in whom a specific diagnosis was made might belong to a higher risk group and might have experienced even higher mortality if they were undiagnosed or inappropriately treated (Fishman, 1979). In fact, some studies have suggested lower mortality rates in patients who had a specific diagnosis established in contrast to those who did not (Greenman et al., 1975; Pennington and Feldman, 1977). A definitive test of this issue would be to randomize patients with diffuse pneumonia into empiric treatment and nontreatment groups and observe the eventual outcome. It is doubtful, however, whether such a study could be executed. Nonspecific "polypharmacy" that might affect most bacterial and parasitic pathogens afflicting the lung is certainly feasible, but reservations about such an approach include: (1) patients with undiagnosed neoplastic or drug-induced lung infiltrates would not be appropriately treated; (2) multiple drugs could interact in ways that could potentiate organ toxicity; and (3) the dosage of empirical and microbial agents may not be adequate or "pushed" with the same confidence than when an infectious etiology is established. In one study, two-thirds of patients having an underlying neoplastic disorder were found to have the same neoplasm responsible for lung infiltrates (Fishman, 1979). Hospital mortality was only 8%, emphasizing the importance of directed radiation and/or chemotherapy in such patients. Thus, in individuals who have an underlying malignant or neoplastic disorder, establishing a specific diagnosis is highly desirable because it would identify alternative therapeutic approaches other than the treatment of pneumocystis infection.

In Hughes' trial of trimethoprim-sulfamethoxazole versus pentamidine in documented pneumocystosis, 40% of the patients did not respond to the regimen to which they were initially randomized. The total of approximately 80% clinical responses included approximately 20% of individuals who were "crossed over" to the alternative regimen (Hughes et al., 1978). It is uncertain if the patients would have improved if they had been maintained on the initial regimen. Equally more important, however, is whether or not there may be differing susceptibilities of *Pneumocystis* strains to the different antimicrobial agents that are available. Without establishing a specific diagnosis of pneumocystis infection, empiric therapy may miss those individuals who could be failing on one regimen and could potentially benefit from an alternative therapy, or identify a group with proven disease in whom the dose of one of the agents could be aggressively increased.

It seems reasonable that an aggressive approach to establishing a diagnosis should be pursued in those patients in whom the underlying disease, such as a neoplasm, has some chance of responding to appropriate therapy. The argument can thereby be advanced that successful treatment of an infectious complication realistically offers better survival. Translated into practical terms, patients who are in a leukemic remission, have an organ transplant that is being well accepted, or have another underlying disease that is likely to be controlled are the prime groups for expending a major effort at establishing a specific diagnosis and basing therapy on that result. On the other hand, empiric therapy may be justified in patients in whom all practical means for treating underlying disease have been exhausted, thus avoiding the added risk of an invasive diagnostic procedure.

Table 5 is a selected summary of published reports using different invasive techniques to diagnose lung infiltrates in patients with impaired host defenses. These studies contain many additional references that may be reviewed. Clearly, some of these procedures are infrequently performed in most medical centers and the enthusiasm about these approaches must be tempered by the fact that the specific authors have gained considerable experience with their own favored approach. There have been a few comparisons of the validity of these approaches in the same patient with procedures simultaneously. One study of interstitial pneumonitis in bone marrow transplant recipients has been reported by Peterson et al. and perhaps gives the best insight into the relative sensitivity and specificity of open lung biopsy versus transbronchoscopic biopsy (Petersen et al., 1978). Both procedures were performed in the same patients under general anesthesia. Of 5 patients shown to have pneumocystis infection of the lung by open-lung biopsy, only 3 had that diagnosis established by concurrent transbronchial biopsy. In the remaining 2 who had transbronchoscopic biopsy specimens, the evaluation was nondiagnostic in 1 and "idiopathic pneumonia" in the other. Thus, it appears that transbronchoscopic biopsy, while more readily performed in most modern medical centers, is not as definitive as open-lung biopsy. One factor underscoring this observation is probably the size of the sample, since relatively small amounts of lung tissue can be obtained by the transbronchoscopic approach.

Of the procedures reviewed in Table 5, our preference is clearly for open-lung biopsy. In the series summarized in Table 3 the most frequent diagnosis was *Pneumocystis carinii* pneumonitis, but many other treatable diseases were found. The principal advantages of open-lung biopsy are that adequate tissue is obtained for histologic stains and culture, the complication rate is low, and potential problems such as pneumothorax and bleeding are usually averted with surgical repair of the biopsy site rather than relying on the lung to seal after puncture. Insertion of a chest tube following open biopsy is "prophylaxis" against sudden respiratory decomposition associated with pneumothorax, which is commonly encountered after transthoracic needle biopsy and transbronchoscopic biopsy. The hazard of open-lung

Table 5 Representative Studies of Different Diagnostic Approaches to Diffuse Pulmonary Infiltrates

Technique	Reference	Complications	Comment
1. Bronchoalveolar lavage	Cauberre et al., 1978; Drew et al., 1974	Rare	Can be performed despite bleeding tendencies (contraindication is severe hypoxia) but yield may not be good as biopsy.
2. Cutting needle biopsy	Zavala and Bedell, 1972	Greater in diffuse disease	For more peripheral "solid" lesions rather than diffuse disease.
3. Fiberoptic bronchoscopy	Feldman et al., 1977; Nishio and Lynch, 1980	Occasional bleeding and pneumothorax if biopsy also performed	Relatively well tolerated but oropharyngeal contamination confuses bacteriologic results. Can obtain washings or biopsy.
4. Open biopsy	(See Table 4)	10% Delayed pneumothorax	Requires general anesthesia. Because of large sample obtained, gives the highest yield.
5. Percutaneous needle aspiration	Chaudhary et al., 1977	Pneumothorax up to 20% of patients	Reliable in diagnosing pneumocystosis in leukemic children, most of whom are in remission. Limited sample obtained.
6. Percutaneous trephine biopsy	Neff, 1972	Pneumothorax in up to 65% of attempts	Limited sample, bleeding may be difficult to control.
7. Transbronchial briopsy (rigid bronchoscope)	Hodgkin et al., 1973	10% Pneumothorax incidence	Use of rigid bronchoscope. Low morbidity but limited samples.
8. Transtracheal aspiration	Lau et al., 1976	Occasional bleeding	A useful initial step in evaluation that "bypasses" oropharyngeal contamination.
9. Transtracheal bronchial brushing	Aisner et al., 1976; George et al., 1978	About 20% of patients have some complication	Limited sample through bronchoscope; may attempt after platelet transfusion.

biopsy is that general anesthesia is necessary and patients probably need to be carefully managed in the immediate postoperative period.

For a patient with a bleeding diathysis that cannot be corrected with an appropriate transfusion therapy, bronchoscopy still may be performed, but the procedure may be limited to bronchial washings and lavage. There are reports that such procedures offer promise, but care should be taken not to instill large volumes of saline, inasmuch as absorbed fluid might contribute to fluid overload. The limited experience of Cauberre et al. (1978) is interesting because it involves using a bronchoscope to "wedge" in a smaller bronchus, followed by lavage. This has been claimed to be successful in a small number of cases and deserved further evaluation. In our experience bronchoscopic washings per se have not been particularly valuable in making the diagnosis of pneumocystis infection, but they may be useful for detecting medically important fungi.

X. Synthesis: A Planned, Integrated Approach to Diagnosis and Management

Recognizing that there may be an institutional or individual expertise with one type of biopsy approach, our current recommendations for the management of patients with suspected pneumocystosis are as follows: It is still appropriate to undertake careful sputum bacteriologic examination in patients from whom an adequate specimen may be obtained. As part of a general evaluation of the immunosuppressed patient with diffuse lung infiltrates, a transtracheal aspiration can be performed in patients whose total platelet count exceeds 40,000 platelets mm^3. It should be made clear, however, that we do not advocate this procedure primarily as a means for diagnosis of *Pneumocystis*. Transtracheal aspiration, which bypasses oropharyngeal flora, may be helpful for diagnosing aerobic and anaerobic bacterial lung infection, mycobacterial disease, and fungal pneumonia. The stain which is used to identify fungi in transtracheal aspirates, the Gomori methemanine silver stain, is the same as that required for identification of *Pneumocystis*. Transtracheal aspiration can thus be a prelude to fiberoptic bronchoscopy. Following transtrachial aspiration antibacterial therapy with broad spectrum agents (a beta-lactam agent plus an aminoglycoside) may be started. Fiberoptic bronchoscopy is now probably one of the most commonly performed procedures for establishing a diagnosis of parenchymal lung disease and many physicians and surgeons are now well trained in the technique. However, during most conventional fiberoptic bronchoscopic procedures, contamination of the lower respiratory passages occurs because the bronchoscope must be passed initially through the oropharynx or the nasopharynx. The use of lavage materials might be also considered in a patient in whom transbroncho-scopic biopsy cannot be performed because of low platelet count.

A realistic perception of the events as they are likely to occur in most hospitals takes into consideration the following scenario: even if the deci-sion is made to proceed with open-lung biopsy it may take several hours to marshall all of the forces required for the undertaking of this procedure (securing consent, scheduling operating room time, contacting a surgeon). In the meantime, sputum examination, transtracheal aspiration, and even fiberoptic bronchoscopy can be performed. With rapid staining methods a preliminary result could be obtained by these procedures before the open-lung biopsy is actually carried out. If a specific microbial etiology of infil-trates is obtained, the open-lung biopsy could then be cancelled. One of the most important principles is, however, that if transtracheal aspiration, fiber-optic bronchoscopy, or bronchial washings yield *negative* results then open-lung biopsy should be undertaken expeditiously before the patient deterior-ates further. As a general principle the chances of survival from any infec-tious process are directly related to the aggressiveness with which the diag-nosis is pursued in the early stages of disease and the early institution of appropriate therapy.

In some centers, particularly with an extensive pediatric experience (Chaudhary et al., 1977), transthoracic percutaneous closed-needle aspiration under fluoroscopic guidance has been carried out without a high rate of com-plications. It may be that in young children lung parenchyma "seals" better after such percutaneous needle biopsy. Our own experience with percutane-ous needle aspiration or biopsy in the immunocompromised adult is that such approaches are associated with an unacceptably high incidence of pneu-mothorax or uncontrolled bleeding, and we no longer recommend these pro-cedures. While patients are being prepared for transtracheal aspirations, fiberoptic bronchoscopy, or endotracheal lung lavage (the diagnostic proce-dures that do not require general anesthesia), we see little harm or danger in giving intravenous furosemide, 100-200 mg. In particular, this should be given to patients in whom congestive heart failure has not been confidently excluded by appropriate catheterization of the pulmonary outflow tract with a Swan-Ganz-type of pulmonary catheter. Intravenous furosemide can lead to dramatic relief of dyspnea within hours and coupled with radiologic im-provement (which may be manifested within a few hours) the more invasive diagnostic procedure of lung biopsy might be postponed or deferred. How-ever, a response to furosemide should not deter a biopsy of the lung if in-filtrates, hypoxia, and dyspnea still persist. The "bottom line" is that if transtracheal aspirations and bronchoscopic procedures do not yield a diag-nosis an open lung biopsy should be undertaken without hesitation.

A team approach is clearly necessary to process any material which is obtained during any of the diagnostic procedures described above. It is frustrating to observe situations in which heroic efforts are expended to obtain consent from patients and/or family, to arrange emergency diagnostic surgery, and to alert specialists about performing laborious studies only to have curcial specimens lost on the way to the microbiology/pathology laboratory or to have the improper stains applied on excellent specimens. To avoid such debacles a systematic procedure must be devised to assign responsibility for delivery of specimens and execution of comprehensive microbiologic and histopathologic studies in an orderly manner.

Many stains have been proposed for identifying both cyst forms and trophozoites. There is little doubt that the definitive stain for recognition of the cyst form is the Gomori methanamine silver stain. New modifications of this technique now permit rapid identification of cysts within approximately a 3-hr period (Ruskin, 1981). In some centers the Giemsa stain has been used to identify trophozoite forms. Similarly, there are some cytopathologists who advocate toluidine blue and rapid Gram-Weigert staining techniques as methods for establishing a preliminary diagnosis (Rosen et al., 1975). Our experience has been that preparations heavily loaded with cyst forms are all positive by the toluidine blue-, Gram-Weigert-, and silver-staining techniques. In samples where the diagnosis may be equivocal, the definitive test is identification of cyst forms by the Gomori silver-staining method.

XI. The Diagnostic and Therapeutic Dilemma of a Nonspecific or Negative Lung Biopsy

A wide variety of pulmonary processes besides *Pneumocystis* may be identified by invasive techniques. For instance, the reported diagnostic yield of flexible fiberoptic bronchoscopy for pulmonary infiltrates in immunocompromised patients has varied 48 to 66% in some series (Nishio and Lynch, 1980). However, according to Nishio and Lynch, the "yield" may be overestimated because some investigators include "nonspecific inflammatory changes" as a diagnosis in itself. Poe and co-workers (1979) established 15 "specific" diagnoses out of 35 transbronchial biopsies, but they included cases of radiation fibrosis and bacterial pneumonia which would not be considered histologically specific. However, bacteriologic cultures obtained through a bronchoscope are of questionable value. Most of the series summarized in Tables 3 and 5 fail to indicate if patients were on antibacterial or anti-pneumocystis therapy at the time of biopsy and the possible effects of such intervention on the results.

Patients with nonspecific changes may recover clinically and roentologically without specific therapy. Some investigators are of the opinion that nonspecific inflammatory changes on transbronchoscopic biopsy are infrequently associated with treatable diseases, but Nishio and Lynch (1980) report that 8 of 15 patients with nonspecific inflammatory changes subsequently had a specific diagnosis established. Two of these patients had pneumocystis pneumonia. In all, alternate procedures led to specific antimortem diagnosis in 7 cases and in 6 of these cases the diagnosis prompted new and specific therapy that resulted in recovery. Thus, in these 6 cases, failure to identify a specific etiology may have led to omission of life-saving therapy and they cautioned against accepting nonspecific histologic changes as definitive. Like ourselves, they advocate open lung biopsy for patients in whom transbronchial biopsy is not diagnostic. If this is not possible, it is our recommendation that patients with nonspecific lung biopsies should be given to an empiric course of treatment with trimethoprim-sulfamethoxazole and erythromycin. The latter is intended to be active against *Legionella pneumophila.*

XII. Sequelae of Pneumocystis Infection

With some of the early studies of pentamidine, postinfection fibrosis was noted (Whitcomb et al., 1970). In rats treated with pentamidine, fibrosis was documented histologically (Frenkel et al., 1966). Children, however, do not appear to develop irreversible changes in pulmonary function (Sanyal et al., 1977). Clearly, patients who developed pneumocystis infection are often receiving other medications which may be toxic to lung tissue, or may develop oxygen toxicity. Our own experience is that some adults with *Pneumocystis* may have persistent lung infiltrates that at autopsy are due to extensive fibrosis. Most of these individuals have an underlying collagen vascular disease or have received lung radiation, alkylating agents, or bleomycin. It has been impossible to assess the relative contributory roles of these factors. The issue of recurrent *Pneumocystis* and prophylaxis is dealt with in Chapter 7.

References

Aisner, J., Kvois, L. K., Sickles, E. A., Schimpff, S. C., and Wiernik, P. H. (1976). Transtracheal selective bronchial brushing for pulmonary infiltrates in patients with cancer. *Chest* **69**:367.

Bale, J. F., Jr., Kern, E. R., Overall, J. C., Jr., and Glasgow, L. A. (1982). Enhanced susceptibility of mice infected with murine cytomegalovirus to intranasal challenge with *Escherichia coli:* Pathogenesis and altered inflammatory response. *J. Infect. Dis.* **145**:525.

Burke, B. A., and Good, R. A. (1973). *Pneumocystis carinii* infection. *Medicine* **52**:23.

Byrd, R. B., and Horn, B. R. (1976). Infection due to *Pneumocystis carinii* simulating lobar bacterial pneumonia. *Chest* **70**:91.

Cauberre, I., Sors, H., and Even, P. (1978). Diagnosis of *Pneumocystis* pneumonia. *New Engl. J. Med.* **298**:13.

Centers for Disease Control (1976). *Pneumocystis carinii* pneumonia in Vietnamese orphans. *Morbid. Mortal. Weekly Rep.* **25**:15.

Centers for Disease Control (1982). *Pneumocystis carinii* pneumonia among persons with hemophilia A. *Morbid. Mortal. Weekly Rep.* **31**:365.

Centers for Disease Control Task Force on Kaposi's sarcoma and opportunistic infections. (1982). Special Report: Epidemiologic aspects of the current outbreak of Kaposi's sarcoma and opportunistic infections. *N. Engl. J. Med.* **306**:248.

Chaudhary, S., Hughes, W. T., Feldman, S., Sanyal, S. K., Coburn, T., Ossi, M., and Cox, F. (1977). Percutaneous transthoracic needle aspiration of the lung. *Am. J. Dis. Child.* **131**:902.

Cross, A. S., and Steigbigel, R. T. (1974). *Pneumocystis carinii* pneumonia presenting as localized nodular densities. *N. Engl. J. Med.* **291**:831.

Dee, P., Winn, W., and McKee, K. (1979). *Pneumocystis carinii* infection of the lung: Radiologic and pathologic correlation. *Am. J. Radiol.* **132**: 741.

Doak, P. D., Becroft, D. M., and Harris, E. A. (1973). *Pneumocystis carinii* pneumonia—transplant lung. *Q. J. Med.* **42**:59.

Doppmann, J. L., and Geelhoed, G. W. (1976). Atypical radiographic features in *Pneumocystis carinii* pneumonia. In *Symposium on Pneumocystis carinii infection.* Edited by J. B. Robbins, V. T. DeVita, Jr., and W. Dutz. National Cancer Institute Monograph 43, Bethesda, NIH, USDHEW, p. 89.

Drew, W. L., Finly, T. N., Mintz, L., and Klein, H. Z. (1974). Diagnosis of *Pneumocystis carinii* pneumonia by bronchopulmonary lavage. *JAMA* **230**:713.

Drew, W. L., Mintz, L., Miner, R. C., Sands, M., and Ketterer, B. (1981). Prevalence of cytomegalovirus infection in homosexual men. *J. Infect. Dis.* **143**:188.

Dutz, W. (1970). *Pneumocystis carinii* pneumonia. *Pathol. Ann.* **5**:309.

Dutz, W., Post, C., Vessal, K., and Kohout, E. (1976). Endemic infantile *Pneumocystis carinii* infection. In *Symposium on Pneumocystis carinii Infection.* Edited by J. B. Robbins, V. T. DeVita, Jr., and W. Dutz. National Cancer Institute Monograph 43, Bethesda, NIH, USDHEW, p. 31.

Feldman, N. T., Pennington, J. E., and Ehrie, M. G. (1977). Transbronchial lung biopsy in the compromised host. *JAMA* **238**:1377.

Fishman, N. H. (1979). Discussion. *J. Thorac. Cardiovasc. Surg.* **77**:344.

Forrest, J. V. (1972). Radiographic findings in *Pneumocystis carinii* Pneumonia. *Radiology* **103**:539.

Fossieck, B. E., and Spangnslo, S. V. (1980). *Pneumocystis carinii* pneumonitis in patients with lung cancer. *Chest* **75**:721.

Frenkel, J. K., Good, J. T., and Schultz, J. A. (1966). Latent *Pneumocystis* infection of rats, relapse, and chemotherapy. *Lab. Invest.* **15**:1559.

Friedman, B. A., Wenglin, B. D., Hyland, R. N., and Rifkind, D. (1975). Roentgenographically atypical *Pneumocystis carinii* pneumonia. *Am. Rev. Resp. Dis.* **111**:89.

Gajdusek, D. C. (1957). *Pneumocystis carinii*–etiologic agent of interstitial plasma cell pneumonia of young and premature infants. *Pediatrics* **19**: 543.

George, R. B., Jenkinson, S. G., and Light, R. W. (1978). Fiberoptic bronchoscopy in the diagnosis of pulmonary fungal and nocardial infections. *Chest* **73**:1.

Giebink, G. S., Sholler, L., Keenan, T. P., Franciosi, R. A., and Quie, F. G. (1976). *Pneumocystis carinii* in two Vietnamese refugee infants. *Pediatrics* **58**:115.

Goodell, B., Jacobs, J. B., Powell, R. D., and DeVita, V. T. (1970). *Pneumocystis carinii* in patients with neoplastic disease. *Ann. Int. Med.* **72**: 337.

Gottlieb, M. S., Schroff, R., and Schanker, H. M. (1981). *Pneumocystis carinii* pneumonia and mucosal candidiasis in previously healthy homosexual men: Evidence of a new acquired cellular immunodeficiency. *N. Engl. J. Med.* **301**:1425.

Greenman, R. L., Goodall, P. T., and King, D. (1975). Lung biopsy in immunocompromised hosts. *Am. J. Med.* **59**:488.

Hamilton, J. R., Overall, J. C., Jr., and Glasgow, L. A. (1976). Synergistic effect on mortality in mice with murine cytomegalovirus and *Pseudomonas aeruginosa, Staphylococcus aureus* or *Candida albicans* infection. *Infec. Immun.* **14**:982.

Hendley, J. O., and Weller, T. H. (1971). Activation and transmission in rats of infection with *Pneumocystis*. *Proc. Soc. Exp. Biol. Med.* **137**: 1401.

Hodgkin, J. E., Andersen, H. A., and Rosenow, E. C., III. (1973). Diagnosis of *Pneumocystis carinii* pneumonia by transbronchoscopic lung biopsy. *Chest* **64**:551.

Hughes, W. T. (1982). Natural mode of acquisition for de novo infection with *Pneumocystis carinii*. *J. Infect. Dis.* **145**:842.

Hughes, W. T., Price, R. A., Kim, H. K., Coburn, T. P., Gugsby, D., and Feldman, S. (1973). *Pneumocystis carinii* pneumonitis in children with malignancies. *J. Pediatr.* 82:404.

Hughes, W. T., Price, R. A., Sisko, F., Havron, W. S., Kafatos, A. G., Schonland, M., and Smythe, P. M. (1974). Protein-calorie malnutrition—a host determinant for *Pneumocystis carinii* infection. *Am. J. Dis. Child.* 128:44.

Hughes, W. T., Feldman, S., Aur, R. J. A., Verzosa, M. S., Hustu, H. O., and Simone, J. V. (1975). Intensity of immunosuppressive therapy and the incidence of *Pneumocystis carinii* pneumonitis. *Cancer* 36: 2006.

Hughes, W. T., Feldman, S., Chaudhary, S. C., Ossi, M. J., Cox, F., and Sanyal, S. K. (1978). Comparison of pentamidine isethionate and trimethoprim-sulfamethoxazole in the treatment of *Pneumocystis carinii* pneumonia. *J. Pediatr.* 92:285.

Jaffe, J. P., and Maki, D. G. (1981). Lung biopsy in immunocompromised patients. *Cancer* 48:1144.

Lau, W. K., Young, L. S., and Remington, J. S. (1976). *Pneumocystis carinii* pneumonia. Diagnosis by examination of pulmonary secretions. *JAMA* 236:2399.

Leight, G. S., and Michaelis, L. L. (1978). Open lung biopsy for the diagnosis of acute diffuse pulmonary infiltrates in the immunosuppressed patient. *Chest* 73:477.

Levenson, S. M., Warren, R. D., Richman, S. D., Johnston, G. S., and Chabner, B. A. (1976). Abnormal pulmonary gallium accumulation in *P. carinii* pneumonia. *Radiology* 119:395.

Lim, S. K., Eveland, W. C., and Porter, R. J. (1974). Direct fluorescent-antibody method for the diagnosis of *Pneumocystis carinii* pneumonia from sputum or tracheal aspirates from humans. *Appl. Microbiol.* 27: 144.

Luddy, R. E., Champion, L. A. A., and Schwartz, A. O. (1977). *Pneumocystis carinii* pneumonia with pneumatocoele formation. *Am. J. Dis. Child.* 131:470.

Lyons, H. A., Vinigchaikul, K., and Honnigar, G. R. (1961). *Pneumocystis carinii* pneumonia unassociated with other disease. *Arch. Int. Med.* 108:929.

Masur, H., Michelis, M. A., Greene, J. B., Onarato, I., Stouwe, R. A., Holzman, R. S., Wormser, G., Brettman, L., Lange, M., Murray, H. W., and Cunningham-Rundles, S. (1981). An outbreak of community acquired *Pneumocystis carinii* pneumonia: Initial manifestation of cellular immune dysfunction. *N. Engl. J. Med.* 305:1431.

Meuwissen, J. H. E. T., Tauber, I., Leeuwenberg, A. D. E. M., Beckers, P. J.

A., and Sieben, M. (1977). Parasitologic and serologic observations of infection with *Pneumocystis* in humans. *J. Infect. Dis.* **136**:43.

Neff, T. A. (1972). Percutaneous trephine biopsy of the lung. *Chest* **61**: 18.

Nishio, J. N., and Lynch, J. P. (1980). Fiberoptic bronchoscopy in the immunocompromised host: The significance of a "non specific" transbronchial biopsy. *Am. Rev. Resp. Dis.* **121**:307.

Paldy, L., and Ivady, G. (1976). Roentgenologic diagnosis of interstitial plasma cell pneumonia of infancy. In *Symposium on Pneumocystis carinii Infection.* Edited by J. B. Robbins, V. T. DeVita, Jr., and W. Dutz. National Cancer Institute Monograph 43. Bethesda, NIH, USDHEW, p. 99.

Pennington, J. E., and Feldman, N. T. (1977). Pulmonary infiltrates and fever in patients with hematologic malignancy: Assessment of transbronchial biopsy. *Am. J. Med.* **62**:581.

Perera, D. R., Western, K. A., Johnson, H. D., Johnson, W. W., Schultz, M. G., and Akers, P. V. (1970). *Pneumocystis carinii* pneumonia in a hospital for children. *JAMA* **214**:1074.

Petersen, D. L., Sale, G. E., and Silvestri, R. C. (1978). Open lung biopsy is superior to transbronchial lung biopsy in immunosuppressed patients with interstitial pneumonia. *Am. Rev. Resp. Dis.* **117**:164.

Poe, R. H., Utell, M. J., Israel, R. H., Hall, W. J., and Eshleman, J. D. (1979). Sensitivity and specificity of the nonspecific transbronchial lung biopsy. *Am. Rev. Resp. Dis.* **119**:25.

Rand, K. H., Pollard, R. B., and Merigan, T. C. (1978). Increased pulmonary superinfections in cardiac transplant patients undergoind primary cytomegalovirus infection. *N. Engl. J. Med.* **298**:951.

Rodriguez-Servera, R. J., Altieri, P. I., and Castillo, M. (1976). Unusual roentgenographic manifestations of *Pneumocystis carinii* pneumonia. *Chest* **69**:422.

Rosen, P. P., Martini, N., and Armstrong, D. (1975). *Pneumocystis carinii* pneumonia. Diagnosis by lung biopsy. *Am. J. Med.* **58**:794.

Rossiter, S. J., Miller, D. C., Churg, A. M., Carrington, C. B., and Mark, J. B. (1979). Open lung biopsy in the immunosuppressed patient. Is it really beneficial? *J. Thorac. Cardiovas. Surg.* **77**:338.

Ruebush, T. K., II, Weinstein, R. A., Bachner, R. L., Wolff, D., Bartlett, M., Gonzales-Crussi, F., Sulzer, A. J., and Schultz, M. G. (1978). An outbreak of *Pneumocystis* pneumonia in children with acute lymphocytic leukemia. *Am. J. Dis. Child.* **132**:143.

Ruskin, J. (1981). Parasitic diseases in the compromised host. In *Clinical Approach to Infection in the Compromised Host.* Edited by R. H. Rubin and L. S. Young. New York, Plenum Press, p. 269.

Sanyal, S. K., Avery, T. L., Hughes, W. T., Kumar, M. A. P., and Harris, K. S. (1977). Management of severe respiratory insufficiency due to *Pneumocystis carinii* pneumonitis in immunosuppressed hosts. *Am. Rev. Resp. Dis.* **116**:223.

Sattler, F. R., and Remington, J. S. (1981). Intravenous trimethoprim-sulfamethoxazole therapy for *Pneumocystis carinii* pneumonia. *Am. J. Med.* **70**:1215.

Schultz, M. (1976). Discussion. In *Symposium on Pneumocystis carinii Infection.* Edited by J. B. Robbins, V. T. DeVita, Jr., and W. Dutz. National Cancer Institute Monograph No. 43. Bethesda, NIH, USDHEW, p. 73.

Siegel, R., and Wolson, A. H. (1977). Radiographic manifestations of chronic *Pneumocystis carinii* pneumonia. *Am. J. Roentgenol.* **128**:150.

Siegal, F. P., Lopez, C., Hammer, G. S., Brown, A. E., Jornfeld, S. J., Gold, J., Hassett, J., Hirschmann, S. Z., Cunningham-Rundles, C., Adelsberg, B. R., Parham, D. M., Siegal, M., Cunningham-Rundles, S., and Armstrong, D. (1981). Severe acquired immunodeficiency in male homosexuals, manifested by chronic perianal ulcerative herpes simplex lesions. *N. Engl. J. Med.* **305**:1439.

Singer, C., Armstrong, D., Rosen, P. P., and Schottenfeld, D. (1975). *Pneumocystis carinii* pneumonia: A cluster of eleven cases. *Ann. Int. Med.* **82**:772.

Sirotzky, L., Memoli, V., Roberts, J. L., and Lewis, E. J. (1978). Recurrent *Pneumocystis* pneumonia with normal chest roentgenograms. *JAMA* **240**:1513.

Stagno, S., Brasfield, D. M., Brown, M. B., Cassell, G. H., Pifer, L. L., Whitley, R. J., and Tiller, R. E. (1981). Infant pneumonitis associated with cytomegalovirus, *Chlamydia*, *Pneumocystis* and ureaplasma: A prospective study. *Pediatrics* **68**:322.

Turbiner, E. H., Yeh, S. D. J., Rosen, P. P., Bains, M. S., and Benna, R. S. (1978). Abnormal gallium scintigraphy in *Pneumocystis carinii* pneumonia with a normal chest radiograph. *Radiology* **127**:437.

Vanek, J., and Jirovec, O. (1952). Parasitare pneumoni. "Interstitielle' plasmazell pneumonie der Fru geburten verursach durch *pneumocystic carinii.* *Abl. Bakt. Orig.* **158**:120.

Walzer, P. D., Schultz, M. G., Western K. A., and Robbins, J. B. (1973). *Pneumocystis carinii* pneumonia and primary immune deficiency diseases of infancy and childhood. *J. Pediatr.* **82**:416.

Walzer, P. D., Perl, D. P., Krogstad, D. J., Rawson, P. G., and Schultz, M. G. (1976). *Pneumocystis carinii* pneumonia in the United States: Epidemiologic, diagnostic, and clinical features. In *Symposium on Pneumocystis carinii Infection.* Edited by J. B. Robbins, V. T. DeVita, Jr., and

W. Dutz. Bethesda, U.S. Dept. of Health, Education and Welfare. National Institute of Health, National Cancer Institute Monograph, No. 43, DHEW Publication No. NIH 76:930.

Walzer, P. D., Schnelle, V., Armstrong, D., and Rosen, P. P. (1977). Nude mouse: A new experimental model for *Pneumocystis carinii* infection. *Science* **197**:177.

Watanabe, J. M., Chinchinian, H., Weitz, C., and McIlvanine, S. (1965). *Pneumocystis carinii* pneumonia in a family. *JAMA* **193**:119.

Western, K. A., Perera, D. R., and Schultz, M. G. (1970). Pentamidine isethionate in the treatment of *Pneumocystis carinii* pneumonia. *Ann. Int. Med.* **73**:695.

Whitcomb, M. E., Schwartz, M. I., Charles, M. A., and Larson, P. H. (1970). Interstitial fibrosis after *Pneumocystis carinii* pneumonia. *Ann. Int. Med.* **73**:761.

Zavala, D. C., and Bedell, G. N. (1972). Percutaneous lung biopsy with a cutting needle. *Am. Rev. Resp. Dis.* **106**:186.

7

Treatment and Prevention of *Pneumocystis carinii* Infection

LOWELL S. YOUNG

University of California at Los Angeles
Center for the Health Sciences
Los Angeles, California

I. Introduction: An Overview

Remarkable strides have been made in the treatment of *Pneumocystis carinii* pneumonia, with some recent studies reporting almost 90% response rates to chemotherapeutic intervention (Young, 1982; Sattler and Remington, 1981). Nor surprisingly, however, the early therapeutic approaches to this disease were born of desparation and rooted in empiricism. As reviewed by Ivady and Paldy, a wide variety of medicaments as well as hormones and physical intervention, such as radiation and shortwave therapy, were initially used to stem the progression of this infection (Ivady and Paldy, 1976). Table 1 summarizes some of these measures, all of which appear to be unconvincing in their effect on pneumocystosis.

A major breakthrough in the therapy of pneumocystis infection came in 1958 when Ivady and Paldy reported on the use of pentamidine, stilbamidine, and neostibosan in the therapy of 19 infants with the epidemic form of *Pneumocystis* (Ivady and Paldy, 1958). This experience was further enlarged with a series of 212 cases of pneumocystis pneumonia treated with pentamidine. In this group, it was observed that the mortality rate declined from 50% in untreated infants to 5% or lower (Ivan and Paldy, 1976). While

Table 1 Unsuccessful Forms of Therapy
for Pneumocystis Infection

ACTH
Antimalarials
Atabrine
Bismuth
Estrogens
Formaldehyde aerosol
Hydergine
Mintacal
Neostibosan
Nitrogen mustard
Nystatin
P-oxybenzoic acid
Prednisone
Short-wave therapy
Streptodornase
Streptokinase
Vitamin K_5
X-ray therapy

Source: Ivady and Paldy, 1976.

there is some doubt about the diagnosis of *Pneumocystis* in some of these cases, (the means for diagnosis being serology and tracheal aspiration rather than lung biopsy), this reduction in mortality was impressive and constituted the first really promising treatment of pneumocystis infection. Throughout the 1960s, increasing recognition of human pneumocystis infection led to more widespread therapeutic use of pentamidine. In 1967, the Parasitic Diseases Drug Service of the Centers for Disease Control received approval by the Food and Drug Administration to distribute pentamidine as an experimental agent (Western et al., 1970). About this time, Frenkel and colleagues reported that the combination pyrimethamine and sulfadiazine was effective in treating pneumocystis infection in corticosteroid-treated rats (Frenkel et al., 1966). Only a few patients have been treated with that regimen, but some impressive clinical results have been observed. Further variations on the approach using an antifolate agent plus sulfonamide include the use of pyrimethamine and sulfadoxine for long-term prophylaxis in Iranian orphanages with epidemic pneumocystosis (Dutz et al., 1976). This approach was successful, but there has been little additional published work on this regimen. The more recent pioneering studies of Hughes and colleagues established that fixed combination of trimethoprim-sulfamethoxazole is effective for the prophylaxis and treatment of *Pneumocystis* in rats and humans and this readily available preparation is widely used today (Hughes, 1981).

II. Pentamidine

Pentamidine (as the isethionate, trade name Lomidine) is 4-4′ diamidino diphenoxypentane, dibeta-hydroxy ethanesulfonate. It belongs to the group of aromatic diamidino compounds synthesized in the 1930s as antitrypanosoma-cidal agents. Pentamidine is still a primary treatment for or prevention of African sleeping sickness of Gambiense variety (*Trypanasoma gambinese*) and an invaluable compound for the treatment of leishmania resistant to antimonials. Some members of the diamidine family are noted to have antibacterial, antimalarial, and antifungal properties but with pentamidine this is clinically insignificant.

III. Administration and Dosage

In the United States pentamidine isethionate may be obtained by contacting the Parasitic Disease Drug Service of the Centers for Disease Control or certain satellite stations of the U.S. Public Health Service throughout the continental United States. The only known producer of the compound is May and Baker Ltd. of Dagenham, England. This material is a light, odorless powder in the form of base, which is supplied in 200 mg single-dose ampules for parenteral injection of 2 g multiple dose vials. The smaller vials must be freshly prepared with sterile distilled water, but the multiple dose 2 g vials can be reconstituted and their contents consumed within 7 days if kept refrigerated in the interim. Pentamidine should not be diluted in normal saline because of drug insolubility and it must always be administered parenterally.

The human dose for pneumocystis pneumonia is 4 mg/kg body weight[*] given intramuscularly once a day for 14 days (Table 2), but longer therapy may be necessary for more recalcitrant infections. The total daily dose should probably not exceed 250 mg even for a large patient. Each dose should be dissolved in no more than 3 ml of sterile distilled water in order

---

[*]See Table 2 for dosage change if the pentamidine salt is methane-sulfonate instead of isethionate.

Table 2 Recommended Therapeutic Doses for Treatment of
Pneumocystic carinii Infection

Agent	Dose (mg/kg body weight per day)	Comments
1. Pentamidine isethionate	4 mg/kg/day	As a single dose not to exceed 250 mg/day
methanesulfonate[a]	2.3 mg/kg/day	
2. Pyrimethamine +	1 mg/kg/day	In 3 divided doses
sulfadiazine	70 mg/kg/day	In 4 divided doses
3. Trimethoprim +	20 mg/kg/day	In 3-4 divided doses; prefer I.V. route initially, with reduction in dose by 1/3 after improvement
sulfamethoxazole	100 mg/kg/day	

[a]New preparation available. See Centers for Disease Control, *Morbidity and Mortality Weekly Report* **33**:225 (1984).

to reduce the volume of injection. The multiple-dose vial may be prepared by dissolving 2 g of pentamidine in 10 cc of sterile distilled water; continuous agitation and stirring may be necessary because the material goes into suspension slowly over a matter of 5-10 min. Solutions with slight turbidity or small crystalline remnants may still be given intramuscularly but should not be used for intravenous injections. For very large patients it may be necessary to dissolve the therapeutic dose in a slightly larger volume than 3 ml and give two injections at different sites.

One problem of pentamidine therapy is irritation and sterile abscesses at the site of injection. In clinical situations where intramuscular (i.m.) injections may be hazardous (such as in thrombocytopenic patients or individuals with bleeding diathesis), intravenous administration can be attempted providing the patient is under the constant observation of a physician or in an intensive care unit. The total dose to be administered is dissolved in 10 ml of sterile distilled water and infused by drip or pump infusion over a 30-min period. It is preferable to have either a simultaneous intravenous line with intravenous glucose running, inasmuch as one of the well-known side effects is hypoglycemia. Blood pressure determinations should be made at 5-min intervals during administration of the drug and at half-hour intervals for 3 hr thereafter. If significant hypotension develops, the infusion should be stopped immediately and blood pressure permitted to return to pretreatment level. Resumption of the infusion at half the prior rate may be undertaken if the patient remains clinically stable.

IV. Pharmacology of Pentamidine

Rather limited information is available about the pharmacology of this agent, due to the complex nature of the drug assay procedure. Thus, virtually all studies have been carried out in experimental animals. Pharmacokinetic studies indicate that following I.M. injection pentamidine is deposited in tissues with the greatest concentration in the kidneys (Waalkes and Makulu, 1976). The drug is then gradually eliminated over a period of 10-25 days. Even at 25 days the concentration of pentamidine after a 10 mg/kg body weight dose was still in the range of 5-10 μg/g of tissue in mouse kidneys. The binding of the agent to renal tissue correlates with its most serious toxicity. In the few human patients studied on a regimen of 4 mg/kg body weight given intramuscularly for 10-12 days, plasma levels were low, in the range of 3-5 μg/ml (Waalkes and Makulu, 1976). These levels remained essentially the same throughout each 24-hr dosing interval and did not increase with succeeding days of treatment. Some serum accumulation was noted in patients with azotemia, but the amount excreted in the urine amounted to one-half to two-thirds of the drug in the first 6 hr after administration.

V. Mechanism of Action

Neither the mechanism of action of the agent nor of its toxicity can be inferred from structure/activity relationships and at least four hypotheses have been expounded for its mechanism of action. These studies have not been carried out on cyst forms isolated from human sources or for that matter from experimental disease. Extrapolations from cell cultures or effects on bone marrow could be misleading but there is some evidence that pentamidine (1) antagonizes dihydrofolate reductase as in the manner of better known folate antagonists (Robbins, 1967); (2) inhibits aerobic glycolysis (Goodman and Gilman, 1970); (3) inhibits nucleic acid synthesis (Bornstein and Yarbro, 1970); and (4) impairs the synthesis of macromolecules (Bornstein and Yarbro, 1970).

The suggestion that pentamidine might act as a direct inhibitor of folate metabolism in a manner similar to other compounds used successfully in combination therapy of *Pneumocystis* is intriguing. The initial human observations were that some patients developed megaloblastic bone marrow findings after pentamidine therapy. Nonetheless, Frenkel et al. showed that pretreatment with folinic acid did not influence the therapeutic efficacy of pentamidine in rats affected with *P. carinii* (Frenkel et al., 1966). This is not convincing evidence against an antifolate effect because parasitic organisms such as *Toxoplasma gondii* might lack a receptor or transport mechanism for folinic acid. Definitive studies must therefore await cyst or trophozoite cultivation, or better yet, isolation and characterization of the parasite dihydrofolate acid reductase.

If pentamidine is an inhibitor of dihydrofolate acid reductase, one might speculate about the potential activity of other folate antagonists such as are known to be effective against pneumocystosis. Methotrexate has not been therapeutically successful and patients have certainly developed pneumocystis pneumonia while receiving this compound. The affinity between parasite substrate enzymes and the antimetabolite as well as the half-life of the compound may both be important determinants of clinical effectiveness.

VI. Efficacy of Pentamidine

A tenfold reduction in mortality in pediatric cases occurring in epidemic situations has been reported by numerous investigators (Dutz et al., 1976; Gajdusek, 1957; Ivady and Paldy, 1958, 1976). Clinical responses have usually been apparent 4-7 days after initiation of treatment. As noted in the early therapeutic studies, radiographic improvement was often not demonstrable for weeks or longer. The greatest experience in the United States has been in the treatment of immunosuppressed patients and in the data collated by the U.S. Centers for Disease Control, 42% of all the patients treated with pentamidine and 63% of those treated for 9 or more days recovered (Western et al., 1970). The only comparative trial of pentamidine with other regimens, namely trimethoprim-sulfamethoxazole has demonstrated a response rate approaching 80% if results are calculated by the initial randomization regimen (see below). Some of the patients were treated with trimethoprim-sulfamethoxazole and crossed over to pentamidine or vice versa after failure to improve, but the success rate is calculated by the initial treatment regimen.

VII. Toxicity of Pentamidine

Of patients evaluated by the U.S. Centers for Disease Control, 47% of 404 patients who received pentamidine for either confirmed or suspected *Pneumocystis* experienced an adverse reaction (Walzer et al., 1976). Major side effects of pentamidine have included sterile abscesses, hypoglycemia, azotemia, liver necrosis or hepatic enzyme elevations, and seizures. Minor complications that have been reported include hypocalcemia, pallor, weakness, flushing, perspiration, vomiting, tachycardia, and gastrointestinal symptoms. The incidence of renal dysfunction has been almost 25% and that of liver dysfunction 10%. The information reported by the U.S. Centers for Disease Control involves data derived from case report forms submitted to the Centers on the investigator's initiative following receipt of the compound for use in emergency cases. In all likelihood this represents an underreporting of the incidence of side effects. Still, there appeared to have been at least two cases in which deaths appeared to follow the use of pentamidine per se and could not be linked to pneumocystis infection or underlying disease (Walzer et al., 1976).

VIII. Pyrimethamine Combined With a Sulfonamide

Experimental studies in rats have demonstrated that this combination is effective in the treatment of pneumocystis infection (Frenkel et al., 1966). A few case reports have attested to the clinical efficacy of this combination therapy (Kirby et al., 1971; Whisnant and Buckley, 1976), but no comparisons have been made to other folate antagonist combinations such as trimethoprim-sulfamethoxazole and only a limited comparative study with pentamidine was attempted at the National Cancer Institute (Young and DeVita, 1976). The preliminary experience was that this combination was as effective as pentamidine but only a few patients were treated. The recommended dose for the pyrimethamine component is 1 mg/kg body weight per day in three divided doses with 70 mg/kg body weight sulfadiazine in 3 or 4 divided doses. This regimen can only be used orally.

A variant of this regimen includes pyrimethamine with sulfadoxine, which has been used successfully for antimalarial prophylaxis. This preparation has recently been licensed in the United States for malaria prophylaxis and was effective in obviating epidemic pneumocystis infection in Middle Eastern orphanages (Post et al., 1971). (See Sec. XV.)

IX. Trimethoprim-Sulfamethoxazole
for Pneumocystis Infection

Frenkel and colleagues initially demonstrated the effectiveness of a folate antagonist paired with sulfonamides in the treatment and prevention of pneumocystis infections in the cortisone-treated rat model (Frenkel et al., 1966). Sulfonamides competitively inhibit incorporation of para-aminobenzoic acid into dihydrofolate, while trimethoprim inhibits microbial dihydrofolate reductase. This sequential inhibition of critical steps in purine synthesis results in net inhibition of synthesis of deoxyribonucleic acid. The limited evidence from human clinical trials that sulfadoxine with pyrimethamine was effective in preventing disease (Post et al., 1971) and pyrimethamine plus sulfadiazine could also be therapeutically effective gave encouragement to use the fixed combination of trimethoprim-sulfamethoxazole in the treatment and prevention of *Pneumocystis* in the cortisone-treated rats (Hughes et al., 1974). The latter studies were quite successful and prompted human clinical trials. Based on pharmacologic differences there is actually some expectation that trimethoprim might work better than pyrimethamine because the concentrations of trimethoprim in human lung tissue have been found to be 1.5-3.5 times greater than in serum (Hansen et al., 1973).

The initial human clinical trials with trimethoprim-sulfamethoxazole have come primarily from two centers, St. Jude's Childrens' Research Hospital and the UCLA Center for the Health Sciences. Hughes and colleagues first treated patients with childhood leukemia with two regimens, a low dosage one (10 mg/kg trimethoprim and 50 mg/kg of sulfamethoxazole) and a higher dosage regimen (20 mg/kg trimethoprim and 100 mg/kg sulfamethoxazole) (Hughes et al., 1975). The initial report concluded that the higher dosage was more effective but noted that this dosage was some three times that recommended for the treatment of bacterial infections in humans. Results in a small series of immunocompromised adults, all of whom were given oral doses in a concentration comparable to the higher doses used by Hughes and colleagues were reported from UCLA by Lau and Young (1976).

Hughes and colleagues provided the definitive comparison of trimethoprim-sulfamethoxazole with pentamidine in a randomized controlled prospective study of 50 patients with histologically confirmed disease (Hughes et al., 1978). The basic study design involved initial randomization to treatment with either regimen (trimethoprim-sulfamethoxazole was used in high dosage) and a crossover to the alternative regimen if patients failed to improve in 3 days. Of 24 patients initially given pentamidine, 18 (75%) recovered, but 9 (38%) of these individuals were "crossed-over" to the alternative regimen. Of 26 patients initially treated with trimethoprim-sulfamethoxazole, a total of 20 patients recovered by 9 (35%) patients also required crossover. In all subjects a full 14-day course of therapy was given. It seems clear from these results there were no essential differences in the two regimens and that in childhood leukemia 75% or more of patients should recover. It is interesting, however, that for both pentamidine and trimethoprim-sulfamethoxazole, the median day for normalization of temperatures was day 4, resolution of radiologic changes occurred between the 9th to 12th day, the rise in PCO_2 to 85 mmHg required an average of 8 days for pentamidine and 9 days for trimethoprim-sulfamethoxazole, and normalization of respiratory rate usually occurred after 7-10 days. Thus, the decision to "cross-over" might well be criticized as being too hasty to assess the initial effects of either regimen. In fact (see below) other observers have documented clinical responses if an initial regimen was used for more than 3 days. The point at which clinicians should consider a crossover to alternative therapy remains one of the major clinical dilemmas with either regimen of trimethoprim-sulfamethoxazole of pentamidine. Not unexpectedly, the major clinical difference between pentamidine and trimethoprim-sulfamethoxazole was found to be in the incidence of side effects. In this study by Hughes and colleagues abnormal values for renal function, blood glucose, inflammation in injection sites, as single or combination of abnormalities, occurred in 14 of 15 patients treated with pentamidine alone. In contrast, only one of 17 patients treated with trimethoprim-sulfamethoxazole alone developed any of these abnormalities. Three patients receiving pentamidine developed maculopapular or uriticarial rash while 4 patients receiving trimethoprim-sulfamethoxazole developed such presumed hypersensitivity complications. The studies reported by Hughes et al. in leukemic children used oral dosing exclusively. In the initial studies of the treatment of sdults with oral trimethoprim-sulfamethoxazole reported by Lau and Young, 5 of 8 patients (62%) experienced a clinical and/or microbiologic cure (Lau and Young, 1976). Cases of clinical and microbiolgic failure (persistent *Pneumocystis* at postmortem exam) had serum trimethoprim levels of less than 1.5 μg/ml at 1½ hr following oral medication. Several cases of failure had severe vomiting or paralytic ileus, conditions that would have impaired gastrointestinal absorption of the drug. All patients successfully treated with oral trimethoprim-sulfamethoxazole had postingestion serum trimethoprim levels that exceeded 5.5 μg/ml, but levels lower than this were often observed during the first three days of therapy. Of the 6 patients treated for 9 or more days, 5 or 83% were cured, and in the 6th subject no autopsy was performed to determine whether or not cysts were eradicated from lung parenchyma. Similarly, Hughes and colleagues noted a relationship between blood trimethoprim levels and clinical success (Hughes et al., 1975). Use of trimethoprim alone, however (e.g., in the patient with severe sulfonamide allergy), is not recommended because animal studies fail to show efficacy with this single agent. Neither is there evidence for therapeutic efficacy with a sulfonamide preparation used alone.

The availability of an intravenous preparation of trimethoprim-sulfamethoxazole would obviate the problem of low blood levels secondary to erratic gastrointestinal absorption. This was first used on 12 patients at UCLA who had histologically documented pneumocystis infection (Young, 1982; Winston et al., 1980). The dose, as expressed in terms of the trimethoprim component was 10-15 mg/kg body weight per day. Initially, the lower dose of trimethoprim was used because of the anticipated advantage of the parenteral preparation yielding blood levels roughly twice that obtained with a comparable oral dose. Of the 12 patients, 8 or 67% were felt to be clinically or microbiologically cured, but 2 patients died with rapidly progressing pneumonitis after receiving less than 48 hr of treatment. Three of four failures had rather serious concomitant infections that were a more likely cause of death. The fourth case however, represented a well-documented treatment failure on trimethoprim-sulfamethoxazole. He had cysts found in a repeat lung biopsy after 10 days of i.v. medication, and subsequently was cured on pentamidine. This case and others like it suggest that there may be a small proportion of strains intrinsically resistant to trimethoprim-sulfamethoxazole and the converse is also conceivable. Levels of trimethoprim were consistently above 5 μg/ml and rose on dosage regimens of 10-20 mg/kg body weight per day. Five of the 8 patients responding to intravenous medication became afebrile or experienced a 10 mmHg increase in arterial PO_2 by the fourth day of treatment. Two patients did not respond however until the 6th day of therapy and one patient did not improve until the 9th day. As with children, no serious side effects were observed with i.v. trimethoprim-sulfamethoxazole (Hughes, 1982). Mild neutropenia and thrombocytopenia responding to folinic acid was observed in 1 of 20 patients in the entire UCLA series (Young, 1982; Hughes et al., 1974), but this reaction or maculopapular rash was not sufficiently serious to stop treatment. In the UCLA studies, 80% of individuals treated with i.v. trimethoprim-sulfamethoxazole for more than 4 days have been cured and all achieved postinfusion levels exceeding > 5 μg/ml of trimethoprim. Correspondingly, Sattler and Remington reported an 88% response rate with an initial daily dose of i.v. trimethoprim-sulfamethoxazole of 20 mg/kg body weight, although they published no pharmacokinetic data of any treated patient (Sattler and Remington, 1981).

X. Recommendations for Therapy

Recent reviews indicate that trimethoprim-sulfamethoxazole and pentamidine are probably equivalent in efficacy, but fewer side effects are associated with the former (Young, 1982; Hughes, 1982). In addition, a retrospective review of published cases shows that almost 88% of patients treated with trimethoprim-sulfamethoxazole for 9 or more days survived, in contrast to 63% ultimate survival for those receiving pentamidine for 9 or more days (Young, 1982). Such comparisons are probably unfair, however, since these data do not represent results of simultaneous randomized trials and published experience with pentamidine (excluding the epidemic form of infantile infection) comes mainly from an earlier period when supportive care and therapy of underlying diseases may not have been as effective. In view of the randomized studies of Hughes and colleagues, it would be difficult to prove that any other agent is more effective than maximally tolerated doses of trimethoprim-sulfamethoxazole, providing that the parasite remains susceptible to this regimen (Hughes, 1982). It also appears that early aggressive diagnostic measures and prompt institution of therapy are associated with a greater chance for clinical success.

Our present recommendation is that either the oral or intravenous form of trimethoprim-sulfamethoxazole is the initial therapy of choice. The latter is strongly advised if there is any question about drug absorption. The dose of 20 mg/kg body weight per day in 3 or 4 divided doses is for both routes, with intravenous dosing leading to higher "peak" serum levels. When patients begin to respond to parenteral therapy we would then reduce the dose to 10-15 mg/kg body weight per day and give folinic acid (5-10 mg) if there is a question of bone marrow suppression. Folinic acid can probably be given earlier and does not appear to obviate the therapeutic effect, but it might be simpler to withhold it for a week until a response to treatment of the infection is observed. The oral dose of 20 mg/kg body weight per day should probably be maintained for the duration of therapy. Initiating therapy intravenously, then switching to oral treatment as the patient improves may also be safe and is advisable in some cases (e.g., limited i.v. access). We would treat for a minimum of 10 days, an average of 14 days if the patient improves by day 5, and for a period of up to 21 days if the patient does not initially respond within a week. Routine monitoring of serum levels is probably not necessary in patients treated parenterally with dosages exceeding 15 mg/kg body weight trimethoprim, but may be desirable in those treated orally.

For the patient who is not responding clinically, the issue of when to cross-over to pentamidine is more vexing. We would observe the patient carefully for 5 days, since in our experience 4 days was the median duration until a clinical response was noted, and probably continue treatment another 2 days if the patient is not deteriorating. Some patients have not responded until after a week or more of trimethoprim-sulfamethoxazole. Still, if patients are deteriorating after 5 days or not improving by 7 days, it would probably be prudent to switch to pentamidine. One of the major reasons for apparent lack of clinical or radiological response is the presence of a concomitant infectious process such as cytomegalovirus infection. Obviously, when a simultaneous infection is present, lack of a clinical response cannot be blamed on ineffective anti-pneumocystis medications.

Two unresolved but obviously improtant questions relate to the question of drug resistance and the advisability of starting treatment with a combination of trimethoprim-sulfamethoxazole plus pentamidine. In view of the difficulty of propagating the organism for in vitro tests of susceptibility (and were they to be available if interpreting such tests), it would be difficult to confirm the clinical suspicion of resistance unless large epidemics of "resistant" disease occur. As noted previously, we are aware of individual examples of in vivo resistance to trimethoprim-sulfamethoxazole, but it remains uncertain as to whether most of the clinical failures that are observed represent drug failure in the face of susceptible organisms, drug resistance of the parasite, or clinical failure in the face of markedly impaired host defenses.

Treatment with trimethoprim-sulfamethoxazole combined with pentamidine has as its goal improved therapy, but it is obvious how difficult it would be to design and execute a clinical study to support this hypothesis. Certainly the risk of cumulative toxicity from both individual components would make this the most toxic of all anti-pneumocystis regimens—and probably for little gain in populations where trimethoprim-sulfamethoxazole has worked well, for example in leukemic children in remission. Still, in some patients where the prognosis seems poor (refractory immunodeficiency) there may be indications for such a clinical investigation, but large numbers of cases would be required. Studies of the cortisone-treated rat model of pneumocystis infection do not support an advantage for pentamidine plus trimethoprim-sulfamethoxazole and have been interpreted as suggesting even some in vivo antagonism (Kluge et al., 1978).

XI. Acute Reinstitution of Corticosteroids

While there is no question that corticosteroids predispose to pneumocystis infection, some clinicians have favored reinstitution of steroids for an anti-inflammatory effect in the acute stages of pneumocystis pneumonia. The value of such a measure has been debated (Winston et al., 1980). The effect of steroids in predisposing to pneumocystis infection evolves over many weeks. Short-term, high-dose steroids may limit an inflammatory response and reduce hypoxia while specific anti-pneumocystis chemotherapy is starting to have an effect. By this argument a short course would appear to offer little danger to the host. Unfortunately, there has been no direct assessment of the value of reinstitution of high-dosage steroids at the inception of pneumocystis pneumonia and there is a good possibility that other opportunistic infections of a more acute nature may be exacerbated. The tendency for pneumocystis disease to be associated with bacterial, viral, and fungal opportunistic infections is probably the single best argument for not "pulsing" the patient with steroids at the inception of therapy for pneumocystis infection.

XII. Granulocyte Transfusions

Although the bulk of evidence points towards a mononuclear T-lymphocyte defect predisposing to pneumocystis infection, cases of *Pneumocystis* have been documented complicating chronic granulomatous disease. In one report, a patient failed to respond to trimethoprim-sulfamethoxazole but did defervesce after pentamidine treatment was given. Lung infiltrates persisted, however. This patient had normal cell-mediated and humoral immunity and despite "failing" consecutive courses of trimethoprim-sulfamethoxazole and pentamidine, she finally defervesced and responded clinically after the initiation of both granulocyte transfusions and trimethoprim-sulfamethoxazole (Pederson et al., 1979). It should be noted that granulocyte transfusions may contain T lymphocytes and mononuclear phagocytes and this could have been the basis for improvement. Perhaps the important finding in this case was that the patient had a mediastinal mass which was surgically removed and contained classic cyst forms of the parasite. The use of granulocyte transfusions is expensive and not particularly cost-effective, yet they might be considered if adequate trimethoprim-sulfamethoxazole levels have been achieved and there is failure to respond clinically to anti-pneumocystic chemotherapy.

XIII. Supportive Measures

Important pharmacologic advances have been made in the therapy and prophylaxis of pneumocystis infection. Nonetheless, it must be strongly emphasized that the nature and quality of supportive measures are highly important determinants affecting recovery. If the patients are markedly hypoxic, intubation may be necessary and a tracheostomy performed for prolonged adequate ventilation. Frequent monitoring of blood gases, adjustment of positive end-expiratory pressures, and fluid and electrolyte management mandate that these patients be cared for in specialized centers within the hospital, such as respiratory care units. The use of volume-cycled respirators with positive end-expiratory pressure (PEEP) has now become standard procedure. Some respiratory therapists still use Drinker type respirators which have the theoretical advantage of delivery of continuous negative chest wall pressure for severe respiratory failure (Sanyal et al., 1974, 1977). Besides pneumocystis infection, clinicians need to be wary of concomitant bacterial, viral, and fungal processes. Compulsive management of ventilatory function is necessary to avoid the dangers of oxygen toxicity.

One of the unanswered questions about the management of serious pneumocystis infection is whether or not therapeutic lung lavage can be beneficial. Severe hypoxia appears related to accumulation of dense intra-alveolar exudate and altered ventilation-perfusion relationships. There have been some anecdotal reports that the benefits of lung lavage, particularly by those who have long experience in the technique for the management of pulmonary alveolar proteinosis. However, there has been no extended experience with this approach.

Management of underlying disease and the issue of continuing immuno-suppression has been a matter of considerable debate. Recovery from pneumocystis infection is often related to the ability to control the underlying disease. Thus, control of systemic lupus erythematosus with appropriate corticosteroid therapy is still an important goal while patients are receiving treatment of *Pneumocystis*. Therapy of an underlying neoplasm, such as a lymphoma should continue if the patient is in relapse in order to bring about a more favorable state of host defenses. On the other hand, it must be remembered that many patients who have lymphoma or lymphatic leukemia develop pneumocystosis in remission, and that this is most likely because of reactivation of latent disease. A few scattered reports of "spontaneous" recovery from immunosuppressed hosts have been attributed to a decrease in therapeutic immunosuppression.

Decisions to decrease immunosuppression must logically be based on (1) the outlook for control of the patient's disease, (2) the potential benefit of suddenly decreasing immunosuppression to improve host defenses, and (3) the treatment of a possible "rebound" inflammatory process secondary to reduction in doses of anti-inflammatory agents. One situation where it might be prudent to rapidly diminish the amount of immunosuppression is in the patient who has received a renal transplant. In that situation there always is the "fall-back" measure of hemo- or peritoneal dialysis to support the patient. Unfortunately, in other situations such as hepatic, cardiac, and bone marrow transplantation, there is no ready substitute for the artificial organ function that is so readily available to manage renal failure.

XIV. Patient Isolation

Hospitalized patients who developed pneumocystosis may well be cared for in areas where there are large concentrations of immunosuppressed patients. Because of reports of clustering of this disease, and the difficulty of distinguishing whether these represent person-to-person spread or simultaneous reactivation, patients with suspected or proven pneumocystis infection should be placed in single-room isolation for the first 5 days of treatment. Measures such as hand washing after patient contact should be employed, but mask and gown precautions seem unnecessary. Prophylaxis of medical personnel or healthy contacts is not indicated, but prophylaxis of other high-risk patients in the hospital will depend upon epidemiologic and clinical findings.

XV. Prophylaxis of Pneumocystis Infection

Second attacks of histologically proven diseases have been well documented
and the incidence in one series has been in 15% of leukemic patients treated
previously with pentamidine (Hughes and Johnson, 1971). Pentamidine is
an ineffective and impractical prophylactic agent against pneumocystosis
(Western et al., 1975). The studies of Hughes (1979) in experimental animals and the experience in pediatric patients strongly suggests that the prophylactic efficacy of trimethoprim-sulfamethoxazole persists only during the
period of administration. Thus, eradication of the parasite does not seem
realistic, and patients who have had the infection have a higher risk of re-
crudescent infection, as evidenced by the experience in leukemic children
(Hughes, 1982) and patients with acquired immunodeficiency (Centers for
Disease Control Task Force on Kaposi's Sarcoma and Opportunistic Infections, 1982).

Routine prophylaxis of a high-risk patient population has only been
well studied (randomized controls) in leukemic children with trimethoprim-
sulfamethoxazole and in young orphans with pyrimethamine-sulfadoxine (Post
et al., 1971). Since there have been no controlled studies with the latter
combination in the last 2 decades, it would probably be wise to avoid its
use. Its principle advantage would appear to be long half-life, permitting
weekly or biweekly dosing. The experience with pneumocystosis complicating
lymphactic leukemia is highly variable, even in institutions that use identical
clinical treatment protocols.

A high incidence of pneumocystis infection prompted Hughes and colleagues to initiate a prophylactic study in a group of 160 leukemic children
for two years (Hughes et al., 1977). One-half of these patients received up
to two tablets of trimethoprim-sulfamethoxazole (160 mg of trimethoprim)
on a twice-a-day basis while the others received a placebo control. While no
pneumocystis infection developed in 80 patients who received prophylaxis,
17 or 21% developed proven infection who received placebo (P < 0.01).
After the code was broken in this double blind study, all patients were then
placed on trimethoprim-sulfamethoxazole. Of 786 children with various neoplasms who received prophylaxis, prevention of disease was almost complete
and only one fatality from Stevens-Johnson syndrome was observed (Wilber
et al., 1980). In another study reported by Harris et al., none of 248 pediatric cancer patients who received trimethoprim-sulfamethoxazole developed
Pneumocystis in contrast to 5 of 10 high-risk patients who failed to take
the preparation for a veriety of reasons (Harris et al., 1980). The routine

prophylaxis of patients, irrespective of leukemic remission state seems prudent if the annual incidence in a given population exceeds 5% a year. Duration of this regimen is unsettled, but careful studies have continued beyond 2 years. If chemotherapy is stopped, on supposition that the underlying disease is cured, prophylaxis can be discontinued.

With a "true" infection rate of 42% in patients with severe combined immunodeficiency (SCID syndrome) patients with this syndrome are prime candidates for prophylaxis (Wilber et al., 1980). Appropriate dosing for pediatric patients is best calculated by body surface area methods. The recommended dose is trimethoprim 150 mg/m^2 per day and sulfamethoxazole 750 mg/m^2 per day. It has been well documented in the bone marrow transplant recipient that period of risk can be restricted to a fairly discrete time interval during the period of immunologic reconstitution that lasts between the 30th and 120th day posttransplant (Meyers and Thomas, 1981). Routine trimethoprim-sulfamethoxazole prophylaxis has been given on an intermittent (2 days/week) and continuous basis at doses of 5-7 mg of trimethoprim per day (plus the corresponding amount of sulfamethoxazole). The former method may avoid myelosuppressive activity when methotrexate is also given as prophylaxis against graft-versus-host disease, but both intermittent and continuous methods seem efficacious.

The period of risk in other transplant patients, immunodeficient subjects, and in cancer patients probably relates to the state of underlying disease. If it improves and the need for immunosuppression decreases then prophylaxis is probably unnecessary. Some authorities give trimethoprim-sulfamethoxazole in patients who have evidence for active cytomegalovirus infection, citing the risk of simultaneous pneumocystosis in that setting.

For all patients with a previously documented episode of pneumocystis infection, it has been our policy to give prophylaxis with trimethoprim-sulfamethoxazole at the oral dose of the trimethoprim component of 5-7 mg/kg body weight per day. The duration of prophylaxis has not been critically evaluated but we would recommend maintaining prophylaxis for one year or more unless there is improvement in immunologic function and/or a decrease in therapeutic immunosuppression.

XVI. Other Prophylactic Measures

Hughes and colleagues have tried unsuccessfully to immunize and protect animals with a pneumocystis vaccine but efficacy could not be demonstrated (Hughes et al., 1973).

Gamma globulin preparations have been given to patients who have impaired synthesis of immunoglobulin secondary to a B-cell deficiency. The effectiveness of gamma globulin replacement or supplementation alone, and the quantity required to prevent *Pneumocystis* have never been rigorously investigated. The clinical impression has been that replacement therapy is desirable and probably has an antiparasitic effect (Ivady and Paldy, 1958). Doses of 0.6 ml/kg body weight every 3 weeks are currently recommended in immunodeficient individuals (Hill, 1981).

References

Bornstein, R. S., and Yarbro, J. W. (1970). An evolution of the mechanisms of action of pentamidine isethionate. *J. Surg. Oncol.* **2**:393.

Centers for Disease Control Task Force on Kaposi's Sarcoma and Opportunistic Infections. (1982). Special Report: Epidemiologic aspects of the current outbreak of Kaposi's sarcoma and opportunistic infections. *N. Engl. J. Med.* **306**:248.

DeVita, V. T., Jr. (1976). Discussion. In *Symposium on Pneumocystis carinii Infection.* Edited by J. B. Robbins, V. T. DeVita, and W. Dutz. Bethesda, National Cancer Institute Monograph No. 43, p. 199.

Dutz, W., Post, C., Jennings-Khodadad, E., Fakouhi, T., Kohout, E., and Bandarizadeh, B. (1976). Therapy and prophylaxis of *Pneumocystis carinii* pneumonia. In *Symposium on Pneumocystis carinii Infection.* Edited by J. B. Robbins, V. T. DeVita, Jr., and W. Dutz. Bethesda, National Cancer Institute Monograph No. 43, p. 179.

Frenkel, J. K., Good, J. T., and Schultz, J. A. (1966). Latent pneumocystis infection of rats, relapse and chemotherapy. *Lab. Invest.* **15**:1559.

Gajdusek, D. C. (1957). *Pneumocystis carinii*—etiologic agent of interstitial plasma cell pneumonia of young and premature infants. *Pediatrics* **19**: 543.

Goodman, L. S., and Gilman, A. (1970). *The Pharmacological Basis of Therapeutics*, 4th ed. New York, Macmillan, p. 1146.

Hanson, I., Nielsen, I., and Bertelsen, S. (1973). Trimethoprim in human saliva, bronchial secretion, and lung tissue. *Acta Pharmacol Toxicol.* **32**:337.

Harris, R. E., McCallister, J. A., Allen, S. A., Barton, A. S., and Baehner, R. L. (1980). Prevention of pneumocystis pneumonia. *Am. J. Dis. Child.* **134**:35.

Hill, H. R. (1981). Infections complicating congenital immunodeficiency syndromes. In *Clinical Approach to Infection in the Compromised Host.* Edited by R. H. Rubin and L. S. Young. New York, Plenum Publishing, p. 417.

Hughes, W. T. (1979). Limited effect of trimethoprim-sulfamethoxazole prophylaxis in *Pneumocystis carinii. Antimicrob. Agents Chemother.* **16**:333.

Hughes, W. T. (1981). *Pneumocystis carinii* pneumonia. In *Infection and the Compromised Host.* Edited by J. C. Allen. Baltimore, Williams and Wilkins, p. 91.

Hughes, W. T. (1982). Trimethoprim-sulfamethoxazole therapy for *Pneumocystis carinii* pneumonitis in children. *Rev. Infect. Dis.* **4**:602.

Hughes, W. T., and Johnson, W. W. (1971). Recurrent *Pneumocystis carinii* pneumonia following apparent recovery. *J. Pediatr.* **79**:755.

Hughes, W. T., Feldman, S., and Sanyal, S. K. (1975). Treatment of *Pneumocystis carinii* pneumonitis with trimethoprim/sulfamethoxazole. *Can. Med. Assoc. J.* **112**:475.

Hughes, W. T., Kim, H. K., Price, R. A., and Miller C. (1973). Attempts at prophylaxis for murine *Pneumocystis carinii* pneumonitis. *Curr. Ther. Res.* **15**:581.

Hughes, W. T., McNabb, P. C., Makres, T. D., and Feldman, S. (1974). Efficacy of trimethoprim and sulfamethoxazole in the prevention and treatment of *Pneumocystis carinii* pneumonitis. *Antimicrob. Agents. Chemother.* **5**:289.

Hughes, W. T., Kuhn, S., Chaudhary, S., Feldman, S., Verzosa, M., Aur, R. J. A., Pratt, C., and Eorge, S. L. (1977). Successful Chemoprophylaxis of *Pneumocystis carinii* pneumonitis. *N. Engl. J. Med.* **297**:1419.

Hughes, W. T., Feldman, S., Chaudhary, S. C., Ossi, M. J., Cox, F., and Sanyal, S. K. (1978). Comparison of pentamidine isethionate and trimethoprim-sulfamethoxazole in the treatment of *Pneumocystis carinii* pneumonia. *J. Pediatr.* **92**:285.

Ivady, G., and Paldy, L. (1958). Ein neves behandlung sverfarhren der interstiiellesa plasmazelli gen pneumonie frihgeborener mit funtwertigen stibiom und aromatischen diamidinea. *Monatsschr. Kinderheiled* **106**: 10.

Ivady, G., and Paldy, L. (1976). Treatment of *Pneumocystis carinii* pneumonia in infancy. In *Symposium on Pneumocystis carinii Infection.* Edited by J. B. Robbins, V. T. DeVita, Jr., and W. Dutz. Bethesda, National Cancer Institute Monograph No. 43, p. 201.

Kirby, H. B., Kenamore, B., and Guckian, J. C. (1971). *Pneumocystis carinii* pneumonia treated with pyrimethamine and sulfadiazine. *Ann. Int. Med.* **75**:505.

Kluge, R. M., Spaulding, D. M., and Spain, J. A. (1978). Combination of pentamidine and trimethoprim-sulfamethoxazole in the therapy of *Pneumocystis carinii* pneumonia in rats. *Antimicrob. Agents Chemother.* **13**:975.

Lau, W. K., and Young, L. S. (1976). Trimethoprim-sulfamethoxazole treatment of *pneumocystis carinii* pneumonia in adults. *N. Engl. J. Med.* **295**:716.

Leggiadro, R. J., Winkelstein, J. A., and Hughes, W. T. (1981). Prevalence of *Pneumocystis carinii* pneumonitis in severe combined immunodeficiency. *J. Pediatr.* **99**:96.

Meyers, J. D., and Thomas, E. D. (1981). Infection complicating bone marrow transplantation. In *Clinical Approach to Infection in the Compromised Host.* Edited by R. H. Rubin and L. S. Young. New York, Plenum Publishing, p. 507.

Pedersen, F. K., Johansen, K. S., Rosenkvist, J., Tygstrup, I., and Valerius, N. H. (1979). Refractory *Pneumocystis carinii* infection in chronic granulomatous disease: Successful treatment with granulocytes. *Pediatrics* **64**:935.

Post, C., Fakonghi, T., Dutz, W., Bandarizadeh, B., and Kohout, E. E. (1971). Prophylaxis of epidemic infantile pneumocystosis with a 20:1 sulfadoxine and pyrimethamine combination. *Curr. Ther. Res.* **13**:273.

Robbins, J. B. (1967). *Pneumocystis carinii* pneumonitis—a review. *Pediatr. Res.* **1**:131.

Sanyal, S. K., McGaw, D., Hughes, W. T., Harris, K. S., and Rogers, R. N. (1974). Continuous negative chest wall pressure as therapy of severe respiratory distress in an older child. *J. Pediatr.* **85**:230.

Sanyal, S. K., Avery, T. L., Hughes, W. T., Kumar, M. A. P., and Harris, K. S. (1977). Management of severe respiratory insufficiency due to *Pneumocystis carinii* pneumonitis in immunosuppressed hosts. *Am. Rev. Resp. Dis.* **116**:223.

Sattler, F. R., and Remington, J. S. (1981). Intravenous trimethoprim-sulfamethoxazole therapy for *Pneumocystis carinii* pneumonia. *Am. J. Med.* **70**:1215.

Waalkes, T. P., and Makulu, D. R. (1976). Pharmacologic aspects of pentamidine. In *Symposium on Pneumocystis carinii Infection.* Edited by J. B. Robbins, V. T. DeVita, Jr., and W. Dutz. Bethesda, National Cancer Institute Monograph No. 43, p. 171.

Walzer, P. D., Perl, D. P., Krogstad, D. J., Rawson, P. G., and Schultz, M. G. (1976). *Pneumocystis carinii* pneumonia in the United States: Epidemiologic, diagnostic and clinical features. In *Symposium on Pneumocystis carinii Infection.* Edited by J. B. Robbins, V. T. DeVita, Jr., and W. Dutz. Bethesda, National Cancer Institute Monograph No. 43, p. 55.

Western, K. A., Norman, L., and Kaufmann, A. G. (1975). Failure of pentamidine isethionate to provide chemoprophylaxis against *Pneumocystis carinii* infection in rats. *J. Infect. Dis.* **131**:273.

Western, K. A., Perera, D. R., and Schultz, M. G. (1970). Pentamidine isethionate in the treatment of *Pneumocystis carinii* pneumonia. *Ann. Int. Med.* **73**:695.

Whisnant, J. K., and Buckley, R. H. (1976). Successful pyrimethamine-sulfadiazine therapy of pneumocystis pneumonia in infants with x-linked immunodeficiency with hyper IgM. In *Symposium on Pneumocystis carinii Infection.* Edited by J. B. Robbins, V. T. DeVita, Jr., and W. Dutz. Bethesda, National Cancer Institute Monograph No. 43, p. 211.

Wilber, R. B., Feldman, S., Malone, W., Ryan, R., Aur, R. J. A., and Hughes, R. T. (1980). Chemoprophylaxis for *Pneumocystis carinii* pneumonitis. *Am. J. Dis. Child.* **134**:643.

Winston, D. J., Lau, W. K., Gale, R. P., and Young. L. S. (1980). Trimethoprim-sulfamethoxazole for the treatment of *Pneumocystis carinii* pneumonia. *Ann. Int. Med.* **92**:762.

Young, L. S. (1982). Trimethoprim-sulfamethoxazole in the treatment of adults with pneumonia due to *Pneumocystis carinii.* *Rev. Infect. Dis.* **4**:608.

Young, R. C., and DeVita, V. T., Jr. (1976). Treatment of *Pneumocystis carinii* pneumonia. In *Symposium on Pneumocystis carinii Infection.* Edited by J. B. Robbins, V. T. DeVita, Jr., and W. Dutz. Bethesda, National Cancer Institute Monograph No. 43, p. 193.

8

Acquired Immunodeficiency Syndrome (AIDS), Kaposi's Sarcoma, and *Pneumocystis carinii* Pneumonia

PHILLIP C. ZAKOWSKI, MICHAEL S. GOTTLIEB,
and JEROME GROOPMAN*

University of California School of Medicine
Los Angeles, California

I. Introduction

Beginning in late 1978, cases of *Pneumocystis carinii* infection began to appear in individuals with no previously documented immunodeficiency. Initially, individual cases seen at various medical centers were viewed as medical curiosities, but in the ensuing months, clusters of cases began to appear. The first detailed report of the association between *Pneumocystis carinii*, a variety of other opportunistic infections, and Kaposi's sarcoma appeared in *Morbidity and Mortality Weekly Report* (published by the U.S. Centers for Disease Control) in the Spring of 1981 (Centers for Disease Control, 1981). A prominent feature described in this initial report was that most of the individuals presenting with this syndrome were homosexually active men. More detailed reports of cases of this syndrome appeared in a series of papers published in December 1981 (Gottlieb et al., 1981; Masur et al., 1981; Siegal et al., 1981). The characteristics of the syndrome as outlined in these studies provide a framework for the discussion of an unusual, fascinating symptom complex in which *P. carinii* pneumonia appears to be the most common serious infection.

The definition of acquired immunodeficiency syndrome (AIDS) is still evolving. The Centers for Disease Control define AIDS as a case of serious

---

*Present affiliation: Harvard University School of Medicine and New England Deaconess Hospital, Boston, Massachusetts.

opportunistic infection or Kaposi's sarcoma (KS) in a patient 60 years of age or younger who has no previously known predisposition to these disorders and is not receiving immunosuppressive therapy (Centers for Disease Control, 1982a). However, besides KS, other neoplasms have been observed in this setting, notably non-Hodgkin's lymphoma, Hodgkin's disease, lymphoma resembling African Burkitt's, and squamous carcinoma of the oral cavities. Some patients do not have *Pneumocystis* or Kaposi's sarcoma initially, but qualify as cases of AIDS on the basis of other intracellular opportunistic infections which are usually multiple and often recurrent. Most all of the microbial pathogens are intracellular, in which cell-mediated immune responses are considered the bulwark of host defenses. One group of patients presents with several weeks or months of FUO, malaise, weight loss, anorexia, and diarrhea of uncommon etiology followed by *Pneumocystis,* other opportunistic infection, or KS. Another large group, primarily homosexual, present with multifocal KS in the absence of systemic symptoms or opportunistic infections. However, many KS patients ultimately develop opportunistic infections spontaneously or during chemotherapy. Initial laboratory tests performed on these patients reveal a wide variety of immunologic abnormalities including cutaneous anergy and a markedly decreased percentage and absolute number of T-lymphocyte helper cells. The latter abnormality leads to markedly low ratios of cells in the T-helper to T-suppressor cells derived phenotypically with monoclonal antibodies.

As more and more patients have been studied in clinics, it has become appreciated that milder symptoms accompanied by similar immunological abnormalities may precede overt AIDS. That is to say, some individuals in high-risk groups with unexplained lymphadenopathy, slight weight loss, low-grade fevers, night sweats and T-helper cell abnormalities have been found to develop Kaposi's sarcoma, pneumocystis pneumonia, or other opportunistic infections. This syndrome was recently termed the AIDS-related symptom complex. By the same token, some individuals surviving pneumocystis infection have gone on to develop neoplastic processes.

The initial reports emphasized different aspects of the syndrome. Gottlieb and colleagues at UCLA presented information documenting underlying immune deficiency and linking the syndrome to Kaposi's sarcoma, mucosal candidiasis, and *Pneumocystis carinii* pneumonia in homosexually active men (Gottlieb et al., 1981). Siegal and associates stressed the high incidence of chronic invasive and ulcerative genital herpes simplex infections (Siegal et al., 1981). Masur and colleagues noted the disease primarily in intravenous drug abusers, some of whom were women (Masur et al., 1981). Taken as a whole, however, the pattern of opportunistic infections including *Pneumocystis* has been relatively consistent. The same may be said for the immunologic abnormalities that have been documented. As patients with AIDS syndrome have been followed, it is clear that the immunologic abnormalities improve rarely, if ever, and that there are few survivors beyond two years after the diagnosis of the syndrome when accompanied by opportunistic infection.

Epidemiologically, the numbers of cases collated in the United States by the Centers for Disease Control had exceeded 1900 by the summer of 1982 (Centers for Disease Control, 1983b). While some 90% of the initial cases occurred in homosexually active men, 27% of cases nationally have occurred in heterosexual individuals. This is a regional variation, however, with 90% of cases in homosexuals in California. While there are major clusters among homosexuals in major cities such as New York, Los Angeles, and San Francisco, other epidemiologic patterns have emerged. These include individuals who have received factor VIII concentrate for prophylaxis and management of hemophilia, recipients of whole blood transfusions and platelets, children of patients who are intravenous drug abusers with evidence of AIDS, and female sexual partners of AIDS patients. A particularly interesting group has been Haitians diagnosed both in Haiti and refugees (children and adults) in the United States and Canada. Recent European cases of AIDS with opportunistic infections include individuals from central Africa who were not homosexual and had not visited the United States, an intrigueing development. AIDS has been reported in more than two dozen foreign countries with the likelihood of continued spread. Much speculation has concerned the etiology of this process, but what can be agreed upon is that the epidemiology of this disorder so far has most closely paralleled that of hepatitis B.

II. Major Clinical Findings in the Acquired Immunodeficiency Syndrome

Table 1 summarizes the major clinical findings associated with AIDS. The symptoms listed, namely weight loss, malaise, low-grade fever, nonspecific diarrhea, are by no means specific, but should prompt inclusion of AIDS in the differential diagnosis when the individual is a member of one of the groups at increased risk. The afflicted populations, summarized in Table 2 include homosexually active men, intravenous drug abusers, Haitian refugees and their offspring, offspring of individuals with AIDS, hemophiliacs receiving factor VIII concentrate, and an increasing number of heterosexual patients who have had contact with bisexual partners. The available epidemiologic studies do not indicate an association of AIDS with specific sexual practices. Denied intravenous drug abuse may, in some cases, explain the transmission of the syndrome to individuals who have staunchly denied homosexual behavior, however, 6% of cases at present lie outside the identified high-risk

Table 1 AIDS Clinical Symptoms

Lymphadenopathy

Weight loss

Fever

Sweats

Diarrhea

Alopecia

Table 2 The Progression of an Epidemic: Types of Patients Developing **AIDS**

Homosexual males

Bisexual males

Intravenous drug abusers

Haitians in the United States and Haiti

Hemophiliacs receiving factor VIII concentrate

Recipients of transfusions, including platelets and whole blood

Heterosexual partners of cases of **AIDS**

Offspring of patients with **AIDS**

Black Africans

Prisoners

groups. Patients will almost always report that they have been previously in good health and have noted no increased susceptibility to infection.

The laboratory abnormalities summarized in Table 3 focus on T-cell-related immune function. As more patients have been studied, particularly individuals with a homosexual lifestyle, these abnormalities have become increasingly more prevalent. Another group that has been carefully studied are hemophiliacs who regularly receive factor VIII concentrate. Approximately half of the patients in this category studied thus far have abnormalities in proportions of circulating T cells (Menitore et al., 1983). The strongest evidence that the immunodeficiency can be progressive is based on our observation in a few patients in high-risk groups (e.g., male homosexuals) who presented with the AIDS-related symptom complex. In the ensuing months T-cell subset studies showed progressive deterioration associated with the on-

Table 3 Laboratory Abnormalities in AIDS

Cellular

  Skin test anergy

  Lymphopenia (reduced total T cells)

  T helper (Th) subpopulation decreased percentage and numbers

  T suppressor (Ts)/cytotoxic subpopulation increased percentage and variable numbers

  Reduced Th:Ts ratio

  Reduced T-cell proliferative responses to mitogens and antigens

Humoral

  Normal B cell numbers

  Increased serum IgA and IgG

---

set of opportunistic infections. The exact risk of progression remains unclear as are the factors which influence progression.

It may be helpful to briefly review the basis for the immunological laboratory studies. The recent development of monoclonal antibodies directed against lymphocyte surface antigens has led to the availability of these immunologic reagents for the phenotypic identification (T helper or T suppressor/cytotoxic) of these lymphocytes. The most widely used of these reagents are the OKT and Leu antisera. Anti-OKT 4 or Leu 3 antibody identifies a population of T cells enriched for helper or inducer functional activity and anti-OKT 8 or Leu 2 the suppressor/cytotoxic lymphocyte population. In patients with AIDS, the ratio of T-helper/suppressor cells in characteristically reduced or inverted in the range of 0.6 or less when the ratio in normal individuals exceeds 1.7. Identification of lymphocytes by monoclonal antibody typing is a definite immunologic abnormality, but is not diagnostic of AIDS. It is important to remember that in the acute stages of many viral infections, such as infectious mononucleosis and varicella zoster, a reversal of helper to suppressor cell ratios is observed. In the case of AIDS, this appears to be an absolute decrease in the helper population rather than an increase in the suppressor T-cell pool noted in common viral infections. Characteristically in AIDS these abnormalities persist, while in most viral infections they resolve over weeks to months. What is clear, however, is that tests of lymphocyte stimulation in AIDS patients using reagents such as pokeweed mitogen or phytohemagglutinin, stimulatory ratios are usually one-third to one-fifth of normal control values. The clinical correlate of these abnormalities is complete anergy which is evident with commonly used intradermal test antigens such as mumps, *Candida,* PPD, tetanus, and DNCB.

III. Kaposi's Sarcoma

This neoplastic condition was first described by the Hungarian dermatologist, Moritz Kaposi, more than 100 years ago. The first description was of an indolent neoplastic process characterized as "multiple idiopathic sarcoma of skin." Nonetheless, the neoplastic process bearing this appellation must be seriously questioned as a sarcomatous process. The Kaposi syndrome that is observed in association with AIDS is far from indolent and usually pursues a progressive course ending in death from infection or disseminated tumor with pulmonary involvement.

Histopathologically, Kaposi's sarcoma is believed to originate in the mid-dermis and then extend to the epidermis. True metastatic lesions have been commonly observed and a multifocal origin has been postulated. As mentioned previously, the sarcomatous nature of this process has been doubted by many histopathologists and the precise neoplastic cell has not been characterized with certainty. Microscopic features include spindle cells and vascular structures intertwined in a network of collagen fibrils. Vascular endothelial cells and a totipotential mesenchymal cell (the latter capable of differentiating into fibroblasts, smooth muscle cells, and myofibroblasts) have been proposed as the malignant progenitor cell. Of interest is that factor VIII antigen, a specific marker of endothelial cells, has been demonstrated in biopsies of Kaposi's sarcoma. Thus, it has been inferred that the presence of factor VIII antigen links or establishes the endothelial cell origin of Kaposi's sarcoma.

The classic form of Kaposi's recognized in Central Europe and in the Western hemisphere is a neoplastic process occurring primarily in elderly men of Jewish or Italian ancestry. Overall, the incidence of the classic form has been quite low. These data exclude the cases that have recently occurred in association with AIDS. Outside of the cases studied in Europe and North America, Kaposi's sarcoma has been endemic in equatorial Africa, comprising up to 10% of all malignancies in Uganda and Kenya. In Africa, the geographic distribution of the neoplasm specifically resembles that of Burkitt's lymphoma, a neoplastic process also epidemiologically linked to a viral infection. An interesting finding in all geographical locations is that the occurrence of Kaposi's sarcoma is some 10 to 15 times more frequent in males than in females. In the United States and Western Europe, there have been several important associations between Kaposi's sarcoma, immunodeficiency states, and lymphoproliferative disorders even before the appearance of AIDS. Some renal transplant patients, who have usually received large doses of corticosteroids and antimetabolites (azathioprine) have shown a high incidence of Kaposi's sarcoma. It is of interest that renal transplant recipients commonly shed cytomegalovirus, an agent which has been associated with KS. Patients with malignancies of the lymphoid system are usually immunodeficient and have a higher incidence of concurrent Kaposi's sarcoma or have developed Kaposi's as a late event. The processes that have been associated with Kaposi's sarcoma have been Hodgkin's and non-Hodgkin's lymphoma, thymoma, multiple myeloma, and angioimmunoblastic lymphadenopathy. Additionally, some patients with Kaposi's sarcoma initially diagnosed and treated as such in Europe and North America have developed a lymphoma.

IV. Clinical Findings of Kaposi's Sarcoma

The clinical finding of Kaposi's sarcoma has been related to the particular geographical and epidemiologic setting in which it has occurred. In the classic form of disease the most common sites of involvement have been the cutaneous areas of the lower extremities, particularly the feet. In AIDS patients, lesions have been observed in many deep organ sites besides the skin and mucous membranes. Included in the mucous membrane manifestations have been the oropharyngeal infiltrates that begin as plaques and rapidly enlarge. In the AIDS patient this has almost always been a poor prognostic sign. Edema is a common feature of the cutaneous lesions and reflects tumor metastasis into deep lymphatics and veins. Dermal lesions, which often appear to be rather benign, erythematous, or faintly bluish plaques may eventually ulcerate or fungate. Superficially, lesions may spread along superficial veins and may be misinterpreted as evidence of thrombophlebitis. Deepseated involvement includes lymph nodes, large and small intestine, and lung lesions where large tumor nodules have now repeatedly been observed.

    There has been no uniform agreement about a classification scheme for Kaposi's sarcoma. Most histopathologists accept the concept that there are four major forms of the disease. These are summarized in Table 4. The nodular clinical type of involvement is usually a slowly progressive form manifested by the presence of reddish-violet nodular or plaquelike skin lesions often associated with edema. The florid form of Kaposi's sarcoma is usually very aggressive and includes the dermal lesions that can fungate. The infiltrative form of Kaposi's sarcoma involves penetration of the tumor into soft tissue with occasional bone involvement. The childhood or generalized form is a lymphadenopathic manifestation of Kaposi's sarcoma. Dissemination occurs early and is particularly aggressive. Skin lesions may or may not be

Table 4 Classification of Kaposi's Sarcoma

Type	Course	Major skin lesion	Lymph node/visceral involvement
Nodular	Indolent	Nodule, plaque	Rare
Florid	Aggressive locally	Exophytic, fungating	Rare
Infiltrative	Aggressive locally	Diffuse, infiltrating	Rare
Lymphadenopathic	Aggressive widely	Rare; if present, any of four types	Occurs

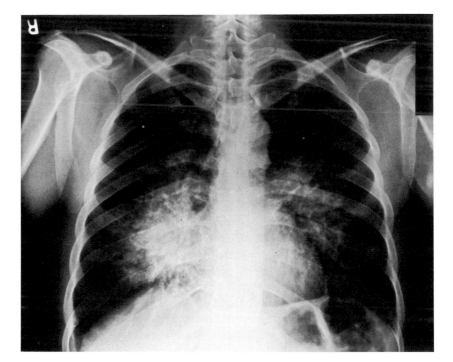

(a)

Figure 1

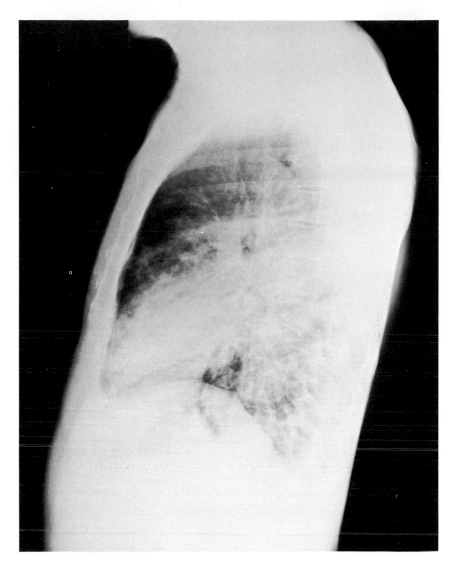

(b)

Figure 1 Chest radiograph of 36-year-old homosexual patient with biopsy-proven pulmonary Kaposi's sarcoma. (a) A-P view. (b) Lateral view.

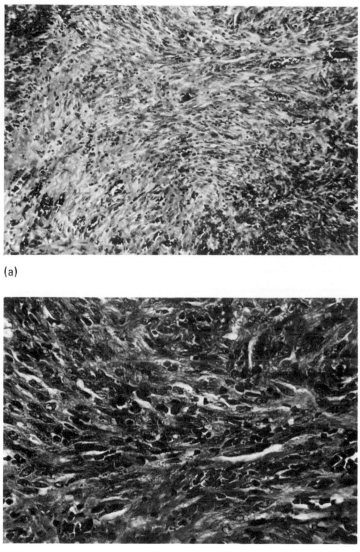

(a)

(b)

Figure 2 Open-lung biopsy of Kaposi's sarcoma from patient in Figure 1.
(a) ×125; (b) ×313.

present and there is usually involvement of the deep lymph nodes, liver and spleen, and occasionally the gastrointestinal tract. The histopathology of the lymphadenopathic Kaposi's sarcoma is similar to that occurring on the skin. Prior to the AIDS epidemic, the generalized pattern was most commonly observed in male African children under 10 years of age. Initial presentation was diffuse lymphadenopathy and the neoplastic process progressed rapidly unless treated. In contrast, Kaposi's sarcoma in older, non-African subjects is quite different. It is not uncommon for an average survival time of 10 years and visceral involvement is much less common. Occasionally, some spontaneous remission of disease has been noted in European and American patients with the "classic" form, some of whom have survived up to 50 years after the documentation of the neoplasm. In contrast, patients with AIDS and KS usually experience the fulminant form of disease with involvement of lymph nodes, lung, and viscera, analogous to that which has been observed in African children (see Figs. 1 and 2).

V. Pathogenesis of Kaposi's Sarcoma

There has been intense speculation regarding the role of viral infection preceding the development of neoplastic processes. The geographic distribution of Kaposi's sarcoma in Africa has paralleled that of Burkitt's lymphoma, a neoplasm closely linked to infection with the Epstein-Barr virus. The high prevalence of Kaposi's sarcoma in similar regions of Africa has triggered speculation that Kaposi's too is a viral-related neoplasm. A human retrovirus (an RNA virus) has been noted in neoplastic cell lines cultivated from several patients with T-cell leukemia (Japan). Development of hepatocellular carcinoma appears in association with hepatitis B infection in some well-documented instances. Impressive evidence has also been gathered implicating cytomegalovirus (CMV) in the pathogenesis of Kaposi's sarcoma. Giraldo and associates observed herpes-type viral particles in cell lines derived from African patients with Kaposi's sarcoma. Serologic evidence of an elevated prevalence in high-titered antibody to CMV has been observed in European and North American patients who have had Kaposi's. Human CMV has oncogenic potential as evidenced by its ability to transform hamster cells and BALB 3T3 cells in culture. Cytomegalovirus infection is extraordinarily common among homosexual males as demonstrated by the studies of Drew and associates in San Francisco (Drew et al., 1981). Molecular analysis of Kaposi's sarcoma tissue using whole virus nucleic acid probes has demonstrated integration of CMV genome sequences into cell tumor DNA in approximately 40% of tumors. Thus, it has been hypothesized that Kaposi's cells may contain specific fragments of the viral genome that are necessary for oncogenic transformation.

In man, cytomegalovirus appears capable of at least transiently suppressing T-lymphocyte/mononuclear cell-mediated immunity. Thus, it has been speculated that CMV may contribute to immune deficiency in AIDS and is able to produce malignant transformation in the setting of depressed host immune responses. However, the high background of CMV infections in the homosexual male population has already been pointed out with a high incidence of shedding of the virus in urine and semen suggesting sexual transmission of the agent. Nonetheless, heterosexual patients and recipients of blood transfusions without CMV infections have developed AIDS. However, most of those patients have had opportunistic infections rather than Kaposi's sarcoma. One extremely important piece of evidence is that restriction endonuclease studies of the CMV isolates from cases of AIDS failed to demonstrate epidemiologic relationship of strains (Huang and Gottlieb, unpublished). Thus, if cytomegalovirus is involved in the pathogenesis, multiple strains would appear to be involved.

Studies have reported a high incidence of HLA type DR-5 in patients with Kaposi's sarcoma (Friedman-Kien et al., 1982). Further studies on a prospective basis are necessary to confirm this association. Certainly the possibility of genetic conditioning favoring the overt manifestations of this neoplasm cannot be readily discarded. There also has been intense speculation that nitrite inhalents taken by homosexuals could result in both immunosuppression and in neoplasms. The best evidence against this hypothesis is that the hemophiliacs, Haitian refugees, and offsprings of AIDS patients have not been exposed to these materials.

VI. Treatment of Kaposi's Sarcoma

Different therapeutic results have been observed depending upon the type of population who have developed this tumor. In elderly patients with the more classic forms of Kaposi's, radiotherapy with electron-beam radiation has been the treatment of choice for superficial disease. More deep-seated involvement has been treated with standard nonelectron-beam radiation. With lymphadenopathic spread and visceral involvement combination antineoplastic therapy has been employed. Some of the active agents include the vinca alkaloids, dacarbazine (DTIC), actinomycin D, and ICRF-159 (razoxane). Recent reports indicate efficacy of the experimental chemotherapeutic agent VP-16 in the therapy of KS complicating AIDS. The superiority of a particular combination with respect to antitumor effect and low incidence of complicating opportunistic infections has not been established and further trials are clearly necessary.

Since Kaposi's sarcoma has been linked with acquired immunodeficiency syndrome, the concept of immunotherapy is appealing. Additional immunologic treatment modalities are becoming available since the advent of recombinant DNA technology. These include recombinant DNA-produced interferons, interleukins, and other immunologically active molecules. Interferons, which are lymphokines, are currently being evaluated because of their effects on the immune system as well as potential antiviral and immunoregulatory roles. Some patients have responded to recombinant alpha$_2$ interferon given in doses of 30-50 million units or more. Experience with lower dosage of alpha$_2$ interferon has been disappointing. It is hoped that new chemotherapeutic antiviral, and immunomodulating agents will be able to modify the currently poor prognosis in established AIDS and prevent progression in patient groups at high risk.

VII. *Pneumocystis carinii* Pneumonia

Pneumocystis carinii pneumonia has been, in our experience, the single most important, treatable infectious complication in patients with AIDS. As mentioned previously, serologic studies as well as culture surveys in the major afflicted population, homosexual males, indicate a high prevalence of cytomegalovirus infections (Drew et al., 1981). Nonetheless, the majority of these infections are relatively asymptomatic. The appearance of *Pneumocystis* in patients with AIDS has varied from acute fulminating illness to a more indolent clinical course accompanied by significant prodromal symptoms of weight loss, fever, lymphadenopathy, and diarrhea.

Table 5 summarizes the clinical features of 14 cases of *Pneumocystis*

Table 5 Clinical Features of
Pneumocystis carinii in AIDS

Frequent

    Dyspnea

    Fever

    Nonproductive cough

    X-ray infiltrate

    Hypoxemia

    Tachypnea

Rare

    Productive cough

    Chest pain

    Cyanosis

    Pleural effusion

carinii pneumonia that have been histologically confirmed at UCLA in patients with AIDS. During the same period, there have been 9 cases in non-AIDS patients. The findings are not remarkably different than what have appeared in other immunodeficient patients with pneumocystis infection. The most prominent findings have been cough and dyspnea, with a lesser percentage of individuals having fever and relatively few having productive cough. We have observed recurrent disease in three patients studied at this center. The second course of documented *Pneumocystis* was really not remarkably different from the first. Unfortunately, in the interim each patient with AIDS had shown significant overall clinical deterioration. Two other patients were demonstrated to have the organism at postmortem examination after a full course of appropriate therapy. An interesting but unresolved issue is whether these organisms were viable, an issue which cannot be settled because of the unavailability of a reliable culture technique.

The diagnosis in all of our documented cases was made via bronchoscopy with transbronchial biopsy. Either the bronchial washings, brushings, or biopsy were readily positive for pneumocysts upon Gomori methanamine silver staining. Frequently, all specimens obtained were positive. No patient had the diagnosis established by examination of expectorated sputum. This contrasts from our experience and that of others (Meyers and Thomas, 1981) where transbronchial biopsy was a less satisfactory means for establishing a diagnosis of pneumocystis infection than open-lung biopsy. It is possible that the degree of infestation by *Pneumocystis* in the AIDS syndrome is far more severe, hence the readily positive samples obtained for silver staining as well as the refractoriness of the clinical infection which we have had to treat. It is our general overall impression that a bronchoscopic procedure or transtracheal aspiration should be the initial diagnostic undertaking; this can be readily performed within a matter of hours and should yield the diagnosis in the great majority of cases. In those individuals who have lung infiltrates that remain undiagnosed by bronchoscopic biopsy, open-lung biopsy should be expeditiously undertaken. There are relatively fewer risks in AIDS patients than in the severely neutropenic, thrombocytopenic cancer patients. Virtually all patients have tolerated one or another diagnostic procedure well.

It is our impression that the therapeutic responses in our patients with AIDS and *Pneumocystis* have been poor, or at least not as satisfactory as in other immunocompromised patients treated with trimethoprim-sulfamethoxazole (TMP/SMZ). Of 14 initial cases, only 8 responded to treatment and were discharged from the hospital. At the time of this writing, only 5 patients are still alive; however, some have died of other opportunistic infections or of Kaposi's sarcoma.

The roentgenographic findings of *Pneumocystis* in AIDS is not dramatically different than in other immunocompromised hosts but can be atypical

(Gamsu et al., 1982; Vanley et al., 1982; McCauley et al., 1982). Although even normal chest radiographs have been reported with documented infection, the most common pattern is a bilateral diffuse homogeneous reticular, granular infiltrate that is usually perihilar and symmetric. These most commonly progress to consolidation, but there can be persistent interstitial disease without consolidation. Occasionally there are nonhomogeneous patchy infiltrates. Rarely pleural effusions are present, although these appear later in the course of the disease. More than one etiologic agent may also be responsible for infiltrates as Figure 3 demonstrates.

All of our patients were initially treated with trimethoprim-sulfamethoxazole unless they had known sulfonamide allergy. Some who were well enough to take oral medication were changed from the parenteral to oral form as soon as clinicians caring for these patients could be reasonably confident of the absorption of the orally administered drug. On the other hand, there have been patients who have been rebiopsied following a period of days on trimethoprim-sulfamethoxazole and evidence for persistent pneumocysts was found. These plus other cases studied here at UCLA in immunocompromised patients (Winston et al., 1980) strongly suggest that some pneumocysts are refractory to the effects of TMP-SMZ. In all fairness, similar phenomena have been observed in patients treated initially with pentamidine—namely that some individuals will respond to TMP-SMZ after the initial course of pentamidine has been unsuccessful. Generally it has been our practice to begin the patient on intravenous TMP-SMZ and to follow the patient carefully in a respiratory intensive care unit setting. Careful management of ventilation and oxygenation as well as the treatment of other opportunistic infections is clearly mandatory. We evaluate these patients every day for response to the regimen, realizing that few patients respond within 72 hr. If the patients do not deteriorate markedly, we would persist in the trial of TMP-SMZ for approximately 6 days before considering a cross-over to pentamidine. Lack of response has usually been an indication to switch to pentamidine, although in several instances the combination of TMP-SMZ plus pentamidine has been used. There has been a striking incidence of cutaneous maculopapular eruptions seen in AIDS patients. Sixteen of 25 patients who received trimethoprim-sulfamethoxazole for documented pneumocystis pneumonia and 8 out of 10 who received it prophylactically have developed a cutaneous reaction (Mitsuyasu et al., 1983).

Several patients that we have followed recently have appeared with cough and dyspnea without abnormal chest x-rays and one patient actually had a fairly normal blood gas of 75 mm O_2. The decision to initiate lung biopsy was based primarily on the severity of the symptoms and the clinical setting suggesting *Pneumocystis carinii* pneumonia. These patients appear to have the best chance of responding through aggressive parenteral therapy with

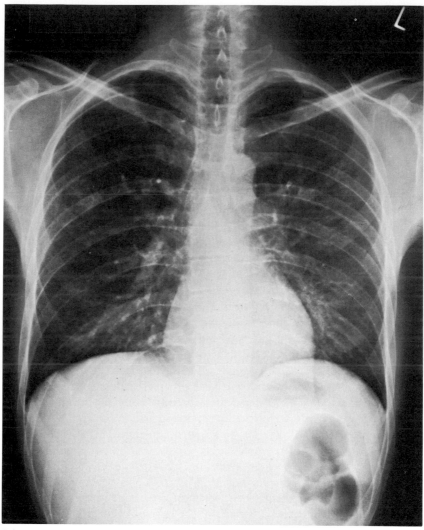

(a)

Figure 3 Progression of interstitial infiltrates over 7 days in patient with biopsy-proven concomitant *Pneumocystis carinii* pneumonia and cytomegalovirus pneumonia. (a) 7/1/83, A-P view. (b) 7/8/83, A-P view.

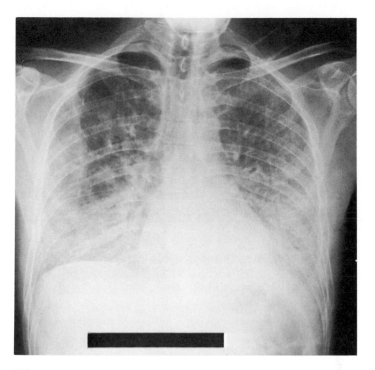

(b)

Figure 3 (continued)

TMP-SMZ. Nonetheless, the possibility that drug resistance is increasing cannot be excluded. Trimethoprim-sulfamethoxazole is widely used throughout the world for a variety of bacterial and parasitic infections and those patients most prone to this complication who are susceptible to the AIDS, male homosexuals, have ready access to such medications. It is conceivable that combination therapy with TMP-SMZ may be more beneficial than pentamidine alone, although this has not been demonstrated in the rat model of disease (Kluge et al., 1978). However, conclusive human clinical trials must be undertaken and are likely to be initiated shortly in which randomized patients will receive TMP-SMZ alone and in combination with pentamidine for biopsy-proven *Pneumocystis.*

Our dosage recommendations for AIDS patients are no different than for other patients with pneumocystis infection complicating severe immuno-deficiency states. 20 mg/kg body weight in terms of trimethoprim and 5 times that quantity in terms of sulfamethoxazole are given intravenously in three divided doses. Such dosing in the presence of normal renal function will insure serum trimethoprim levels in excess of 5 μg/ml, with blood level associated with clinical cure in the vast majority of patients carefully studied to date (Young et al., 1982). The dose of pentamidine (obtained from the U.S. Centers for Disease Control) is 4 mg/kg body weight per day in intra-muscular dose. We believe that some very large patients may tolerate up to 300 mg pentamidine as a single dose or divided into two doses given simul-taneously. However, we would not attempt to give more than 300 mg of this medication in one intramuscular injection due to the problems with sterile abscesses at the site of injection. Based on recent animal data of respiratory transmission, we would suggest respiratory isolation from other AIDS patients and other immunocompromised patients (Hughes, 1983).

Most patients with AIDS who have had documented pneumocystis in-fection have been placed on TMP-SMZ prophylaxis upon discharge from the hospital. Nonetheless, the incidence of recurring infection is fairly high; 4 out of 8 in one early report of recurrent pneumocystis infection from the CDC and in our experience the numbers are 3 out of 14. It is clear from the followup of patients with Kaposi's sarcoma or in male homosexuals with abnormalities of T-lymphocyte reactivity that some of these patients will in-evitably develop *Pneumocystis*. Studies of the efficacy of TMP-SMZ in these populations particularly in comparison with other alternative regimens such as pyrimethamine-sulfidoxine or pyrimethamine-sulfadiazine seem warranted.

VIII. Other Opportunistic Infections

Increasingly, a wide variety of other pathogens are being isolated from pa-tients with AIDS. These are summarized in Table 6 with lists of the appro-priate references in the current medical literature to this problem specifically occurring in the AIDS syndrome. Almost all the pathogens listed are those in which it is believed that the T-cell-mediated mononuclear phagocyte limb of host responses is a crucial component of host defenses. It is remarkable that in the followup of more than 3 dozen seriously ill patients with AIDS hospitalized at UCLA, none has developed an acute pyogenic infection such as pneumococcal, streptococcal, or gram-negative septicemia, unless there was a complication of some nosocomial manipulation such as intubation or cathe-terization. These findings strongly suggest that neutrophil phagocyte re-sponses are entirely normal and are adequate to prevent serious opportunistic

Table 6 Infectious Complications of AIDS

Bacterial

Mycobacterium avium intracellulare: pulmonary, disseminated (Zakowski et al., 1982; Greene et al., 1982)

Mycobacterium tuberculosis: adenitis, pulmonary, disseminated (Vieira et al., 1983; Pitchenik et al., 1983b)

Mycobacterium kansasii: pulmonary (Pitchenik et al., 1983b)

Nocardia sp.: pulmonary (Follansbee et al., 1982)

Legionella sp.: (McCauley et al., 1982)

Fungal

Candida albicans: oroesophageal (Gottlieb et al., 1981)

Cryptococcus neoformans: pulmonary, CNS, disseminated (Follansbee et al., 1982; Mildvan et al., 1982)

Aspergillus sp.: pulmonary (Masur et al., 1982)

Histoplasma capsulatum: disseminated (Small et al., 1983)

Coccidioides immitis: disseminated

Petriellidium boydii: pulmonary

Viral

Cytomegalovirus: disseminated, pulmonary, retinitis, CNS (Gottlieb et al., 1981; Siegal et al., 1981; Holland et al., 1982; Neuwirth et al., 1982; Mildvan et al., 1982)

Herpes simplex: progressive (Siegal et al., 1981)

Varicella-zoster: (Poon et al., 1983; Masur et al., 1981)

Adenovirus: urinary (DeJong et al., 1983)

Progressive multifocal leukoencephalopathy (JC virus): (Miller et al., 1982)

Protozoal

Pneumocystis carinii: pulmonary, ? disseminated (Gottlieb et al., 1981; Follansbee et al., 1982)

Toxoplasma gondii: CNS, pulmonary (Vieira et al., 1983; Pitchenik et al., 1983a, b)

Cryptosporidium: enteritis (Centers for Disease Control, 1982b)

Isospora belli: enteritis (Pitchenik et al., 1983b)

infections that are common in other immunosuppressed states such as leukemia. Perhaps even more significant is the observation that systemic candidiasis has never occurred in our patient population and has been infrequently reported in other patients. The great majority of patients have candidal colonization or infection of mucosal surfaces, esophagitis and severe cutaneous infection, analogous to the chronic mucocutaneous syndrome, but remarkably, systemic candidiasis is uncommon. Also, despite the ready presence of scores of *Aspergillus* species in the environment, aspergillus pneumonia has rarely been documented and mucor infection has not been documented in these patients. Such experiments of nature conferred by the presence of the acquired immunodeficiency state strongly suggest that the neutrophil may thus be the important bulwark of defense against systemic candidiasis, mucormycosis, and aspergillosis.

Several protozoan parasites, other than *Pneumocystis carinii* have been found to infect patients with AIDS more frequently than expected. Taxonomically they are closely related coccidian parasites (suborder Eimerina) and include *Cryptosporidium, Isospora belli* and *Toxoplasma gondii.* Both *Cryptosporodium* and *Isospora* cause enteritis whereas toxoplasmosis has a predilection for the central nervous system.

Although identified in 1907, *Cryptosporidium* has rarely been documented in man, with approximately 12 cases in non-AIDS patients occurring through 1982 (Tzipori, 1983). *Cryptosporidium* is a well-described intestinal pathogen causing diarrhea in many species, calves, lambs, chickens, and guinea pigs among others. Human infestation was considered rare and usually limited to the immunocompromised host. Very recently it has been recognized as a zoonotic disease that can affect normal humans exposed to diseased animals (Current et al., 1983). In the immunocompetent person, cryptosporidiosis manifests as a self-limited, flulike gastrointestinal illness with diarrhea and abdominal cramps lasting from one to ten days. However, in the AIDS patient, cryptosporidiosis is far different. The illness is a chronic profuse watery diarrhea, often of the secretory type. The mean duration of diarrhea is four months, but often lasts until the patient's death. Bowel movements number from 6 to 25 per day with a stool volume of 1 to 17 liters/day. The organisms invade only the microvillus border of epithelial cells and can be demonstrated by histolic examination of biopsy material and demonstration of the 4-5 μ protozoan parasite. Although considered primarily a small bowel parasite, it is now known to infect large bowel and even gallbladder. The mechanism of injury and the subsequent diarrhea is not known. Diagnosis in the past was primarily via biopsy but now with better stool detection techniques this may be unnecessary. The best current techniques appear to involve a three-step stool examination to distinguish *Cryptosporidium* oocysts from yeast cells (Ma and Soave, 1983). These are approximately of the same size and morphology as cryptosporidia oocysts. This entails iodine wet mount for preliminary identification where the oocysts are clear, modified Kinyoun acidfast smear where oocysts stain red, and Sheather's sugar coverslip flotation for concentration of oocysts which then can be examined under high-power objective or by phase contrast microscopy. Although this is an important agent to consider and diagnose in the AIDS patient, there is no reliably effective therapy (Tzipori, 1983; Centers for Disease Control, 1982b). The subsequent diarrhea caused by *Cryptosporidium* has not been a direct cause of death, but the associated malnutrition has often been a contributing factor.

A less frequent reported cause of chronic diarrhea in the AIDS patient is *Isospora belli* (coccidioisis) (Pitchenik et al., 1983b). This organism has been recognized to cause diarrheal disease in humans though it is still an unusual pathogen. In the normal human host the infestation is symptomless or a mild, self-limited diarrhea suggestive of a malabsorptive process. In the AIDS patient this pathogen causes a chronic diarrhea that can last months. There have been fewer case reports of *Isospora* than *Cryptosporidium* so less details of the disease process are known. The diagnosis can be made via stool examination, duodenal "string" test, or by biopsy of the bowel. There is no treatment of proven value, but trimethoprim-sulfamethoxazole has been reported to be of benefit in the non-AIDS patient (Westerman and Christensen, 1979).

Toxoplasma gondii can be considered tissue coccidia and are obligate intracellular parasites. It is acquired by humans primarily by eating meat that contains cysts or via ingestion of cat feces contaminated with oocysts. In normal hosts toxoplasmosis is usually clinically inapparent, but can cause congenital central nervous system infection, lymphadenitis, or uveitis. Infection in the immunocompromised host has a special predilection for the central nervous system (CNS). Neurologic manifestations predominated in more than half of a series of non-AIDS immunocompromised patients (Ruskin, 1981). In the AIDS population most of the reported cases to date are CNS toxoplasmosis. The incidence of toxoplasmosis in Haitian AIDS patients is greater than in other AIDS patients. This probably reflects a higher prevalence of exposure to and past infection with toxoplasmosis among Haitians. The subsequent immunosuppression of AIDS presumably allows reactivation of latent infection. There have been 12 reported cases of CNS toxoplasmosis in 30 reported cases of AIDS in Haitians in two recently reported series (Pitchenik et al., 1983; Vieira et al., 1983). Nine of these patients had focal neurologic deficits with or without seizures and four presented with headache. It appears that computerized tomography will reliably reveal enhancing lesions. The clinical diagnosis in an AIDS patient should be entertained on the basis of neurologic findings and computerized tomographic brain scans. Serologic findings were not always helpful and the IgM was negative in 4 out of 8

patients in one series (Horowitz et al., 1983). Biopsy is the definitive way
to establish the diagnosis. However, identification of *T. gondii* in biopsy
specimens of the CNS has been reported to be difficult because the predominant form was the tachyzoite and not the encysted form. Therapy for toxoplasmosis in the AIDS patient includes the standard regimen of pyrimethamine and sulfadiazine and appears reasonably effective.

Mycobacterial infection is inextricably related to the host's cellular immune system. Consequently it is not surprising to see that patients with
AIDS develop disease due to mycobacteria. However, the extent of disease
and the bacillary load found in AIDS patients with mycobacterial infection
reflects the severity and uniqueness of the cellular immune compromise. *Mycobacterium avium intracellulare* is the predominant organism found to infect
these patients with the exception of the Haitian subpopulation, where *Mycobacterium tuberculosis* predominates (Zakowski et al., 1982; Greene et al.,
1982; Pitchenik et al., 1983b). There have been isolated cases of other
atypical mycobacterial disease.

The organism known as mycobacterial avium-intracellular complex (MAC)
are a group of closely related yet serologically distinct bacteria. MAC belong
to Runyan's group III, the nonphotochromogens. These organisms can infect
many different animals and are relatively ubiquitous in the environment, even
being found in soil, dust, and sea water. Disease in man, though not uncommon, is almost always pulmonary, usually acquired environmentally, and not
transmitted person-to-person. Disseminated infection has been distinctly unusual prior to the AIDS epidemic. In our experience at UCLA, up to June
1983, we have had 21 AIDS patients with documented MAC infection. Nine
of these patients have had positive blood cultures. Usually MAC is disseminated in these patients and has been isolated from sputum, bronchial washings, lung tissue, liver, bone marrow, spleen, urine, intestines, lymph nodes,
brain, and adrenals. The diagnosis should be considered in any febrile AIDS
patient, but especially those who have abnormal liver function tests with or
without hepatomegaly or splenomegaly. Although this may encompass most
patients at one time or another, the diagnosis should always be in the differential and when tissue is obtained for another reason (i.e., bone marrow for
evaluation of cytopenia) it should be processed for acid-fast stain and culture.
There have been several instances of a fortuitous diagnosis of MAC made this
way. Sputum samples and blood cultures are the easiest samples to obtain
and can be diagnostic. One should be sure to instruct the clinical lab to
hold the blood culture bottles for an extended length of time because of the
slow growing nature of the organism. Although blood culture media are being developed that are selective for mycobacteria, in the interim both routine
blood culture bottles and biphasic fungal culture bottles should be used. Bone
marrow biopsies in suspected cases are easy to obtain. Bronchoscopy with

washings and transbronchial biopsy and liver biopsies are worthwhile where appropriate. Histopathologically, even when the tissue specimens are packed with acid-fast organisms by stain there is an amazing paucity of granulomata. This is presumably because an intact cell-mediated immunity is needed for granuloma formation. Although there is some early evidence for a predominance of serotypes 8 and 4 of the MAC strains, our preliminary findings have not substantiated this data (Greene et al., 1982).

Despite being better able to make the diagnosis of MAC infection because of an increased index of suspicion, the therapeutic results are discouraging. In vitro sensitivity studies of patient isolates reveal them to be uniformly resistant to some if not all of the antituberculous drugs. The in vitro sensitivity data are best for two drugs not currently approved for the therapy of MAC: clofazimine, a drug used in the therapy of leprosy, and ansamycin (LM-427), an experimental antimycobacterial drug from Italy. The typical recommended regimen includes isoniazid, rifampin, ethionamide, cycloserine, streptomycin, and ethambutol (Davidson, 1982). Unfortunately, this regimen can be toxic and is not very efficacious, but at this point in time is the best regimen available. The limited trials of clofazimine and ansamycin have not yielded dramatic results and even transfer factor and thymosin fraction 5 have been attempted without success.

Mycobacterium tuberculosis in AIDS patients seems primarily to be seen in the Haitian subpopulation. Although it can manifest as adenitis, *Mycobacterium tuberculosis* usually is miliary or disseminated in nature in these patients. There is one case of brain abscesses caused by *M. tuberculosis*. The tuberculosis infections tended to be the first infection noted in this group whereas this is not usually the case with MAC infection. Diagnosis and therapy are standard for *M. tuberculosis* disease. The higher rate of *M. tuberculosis* in Haitians versus MAC in non-Haitians may merely reflect the higher rate of past exposure and positive skin test status seen in the Haitian population. Presumably the AIDS merely allows reactivation of a latent infection.

The viral infections to which the AIDS patients are susceptible belong primarily to the herpesvirus group. Included in this group are cytomegalovirus, herpes simplex, herpes varicella zoster and Epstein-Barr virus (EBV). Of these, only EBV has clinically not been a problem. However, there have been striking elevations of EBV titers without a mononucleosis type syndrome (Small et al., 1983). Upon closer examination the elevations of EBV titers appear limited to antibodies of the immunoglobulin G class against the viral capsid antigen (Rogers et al., 1983).

Cytomegalovirus (CMV) is strikingly more prevalent among homosexuals than heterosexuals. The prevalence of antibody to CMV is almost 94% among homosexual men but only 54% among heterosexual men (Drew et al., 1981). Although this represents probably past exposure viruria was present in 14% of homosexual men tested. In the AIDS patients, CMV complement fixation titers were significantly higher than for controls, but not by indirect hemagglutination titers (Rogers et al., 1983). Cytomegalovirus was isolated from 25% of AIDS patients via urine and throat specimens versus only 7% of controls. Early in the AIDS epidemic CMV was suggested as an etiologic agent. However DNA restriction endonuclease analysis has revealed different restriction patterns, suggesting that different CMV strains are being isolated from different patients (Rogers et al., 1983). This evidence in conjunction with the known high prevalence of CMV in homosexual men suggests acquisition of CMV in the past, presumably related to sexual activity.

Although CMV is widely prevalent among homosexual men, it usually represents a latent infection that can reactivate with immunosuppression. Unfortunately, this mechanism probably accounts for the occurrence of clinical disease in the AIDS patients. Clinical CMV disease in the AIDS patient usually presents as an interstitial pneumonia, but frequently disseminates and produces positive blood cultures. Involvement of multiple organs has been reported including the retina, brain, adrenals, and gastrointestinal tract (Gottlieb et al., 1983). Therapy for CMV infections in other groups of immunocompromised patients has been attempted with interferon, adenine arabinoside, acyclovir, transfer factor, and hyperimmune globulin among other agents (Ho, 1982). These agents have all met with limited success and at this point there is no reliably effective therapy.

Herpes simplex virus (HSV) infection in the AIDS patient was one of the early described findings (Siegal et al., 1981). Herpes simplex virus is usually seen as chronic perianal ulcerative lesions in the AIDS patient. Fortunately acyclovir is an effective therapy for this problem. Herpes varicella zoster (HVZ) is seen less often than HSV. Acyclovir has been shown to halt progression of HVZ in non-AIDS immunocompromised patients (Balfour et al., 1983) and should also be efficacious in the AIDS patient.

Of the fungal infections seen in AIDS patients, the only one that commonly occurs is oropharyngeal and esophageal candidiasis. Oral candidiasis was one of the original findings and has continued to be a frequent finding (Gottlieb et al., 1981, 1983). Oral candidiasis can often be controlled with nystatin suspension. Esophageal candidiasis can be a more vexing problem and cause severe odynophagia or dysphagia. These complaints in an AIDS patient should prompt endoscopy to document esophagitis due to *Candida* as opposed to other causes. Oral nystatin suspension may be helpful. If unsuccessful ketoconazole or amphotericin B therapy should be utilized (Gottlieb et al., 1983).

Although no etiologic agent has yet been identified, certain precautions can be observed in order to minimize, or perhaps eliminate the risk to health care workers of contracting AIDS (Centers for Disease Control, 1982). Al-

Table 7 Guidelines for Care of Patients with AIDS

1. Avoid accidental wounds from sharp instruments contaminated with potentially infectious material.
2. Avoid contact of open skin lesions with material from AIDS patients.
3. Gloves should be worn when handling blood specimens, blood-soiled items, body fluids, excretions, secretions, as well as materials and objects exposed to them.
4. Gowns should be worn when clothing may be soiled with blood, secretions, excretions, or body fluids.
5. Hands should be washed after removing gowns and gloves and before leaving patient rooms and when contaminated by blood.
6. Blood or other specimens should be labelled "AIDS PRECAUTIONS" and placed in a second container (impervious bag) for transport.
7. Blood spills should be cleaned up promptly with a disinfectant (1:10 dilution of 5.25% sodium hypochlorite).
8. Articles soiled with blood should be placed in an impervious bag labelled "AIDS PRECAUTIONS" and processed accordingly.
9. Disposable needles and syringes are preferred.
10. Needles should be disposed of properly and carefully.
11. A private room is indicated for patients too ill to use good hygiene, altered behavior, or with infections requiring isolation.

Source: Modified from CDC guidelines, Precautions for Clinical Staff (1982).

though care should be exercised in tending to the AIDS patient, one should keep in mind that as yet no AIDS cases have been documented among health care workers caring for these patients. There have been four reported cases in health care personnel, none with documented contact with another AIDS patient (Centers for Disease Control, 1983a). The source of the AIDS in these patients is unclear. The precautions are based upon the epidemiologic data that transmission of the agent appears to require intimate, direct contact involving mucosal surfaces, such as sexual contact or through parenteral spread. Thus, since the mode of spread appears to be similar to hepatitis B infection, the same precautions for hospital personnel caring for patients with AIDS should be observed as those used for patients with hepatitis B infection (Table 7).

The acquired immunodeficiency syndrome is an epidemic with devastating results. The origin and etiology of AIDS is still unknown but investigation of potential causative agents has been undertaken. Until the agent(s) and a potential therapy have been elucidated, the AIDS epidemic probably will continue with the physician, in the interim, relegated to caring for its manifestations. However many clinical and basic science investigators are devoting much time and energy to this vexing problem. Hopefully the answers will be shortly forthcoming.

Note Added in Proof

Since this manuscript was written, substantial evidence has accumulated that the causative agent of AIDS has been isolated. This is the work of investigators in France and the United States:

Barre-Sinoussi, F., Chermann, J. C., Rey, F., Nugeyre, M. T., Chamaret, S., Gruest, J., Daugnet, C., Axler-Blin, C., Vezinet-Brun, F., Rouzioux, C., Rozenbaum, W., and Montagnier, L. (1983). Isolation of a T-Lymphotopic retrovirus from a patient at risk for acquired immune deficiency syndrome (AIDS). *Science* **220**:868-871.
Popovic, M., Sarngadharan, M. G., Read, E., and Gallo, R. C. (1984). Detection, isolation and continuous production of cytopathic retroviruses (HTLV-III) from patients with AIDS and pre-AIDS. *Science* **224**:297-300.

References

Balfour, H. H., Bean, B., Laskin, O. L., Ambinder, R. F., Meyers, J. D., Wade, J. C., Zaia, J. A., Aeppli, D., Kirk, L. E., Segreti, A. C., and Keeney, R. E. (1983). Acyclovir halts progression of herpes zoster in immunocompromised patients. *N. Engl. J. Med.* **308**:1448-1453.
Centers for Disease Control. (1981). Pneumocystis pneumonia—Los Angeles. *Morbid. Mortal. Weekly Rep.* **30**:250-252.
Centers for Disease Control. (1982a). Update on Kaposi's sarcoma and opportunistic infections in previously healthy persons—United States. *Morbid. Mortal. Weekly Rep.* **31**:294-301.
Centers for Disease Control. (1982b). Cryptosporidiosis: Assessment of chemotherapy of males with acquired immunodeficiency syndrome (AIDS). *Morbid. Mortal. Weekly Rep.* **31**:589-592.
Centers for Disease Control. (1982c). Acquired immune deficiency syndrome (AIDS): Precautions for clinical and laboratory staffs. *Morbid. Mortal. Weekly Rep.* **31**:576-580.
Centers for Disease Control. (1983a). An evaluation of the acquired immunodeficiency syndrome (AIDS) reported in health care personnel—U.S. *Morbid. Mortal. Weekly Rep.* **32**:358-360.

Centers for Disease Control. (1983b). Update: Acquired immunodeficiency syndrome (AIDS)–United States. *Morbid. Mortal. Weekly Rep.* **30**:389-391.

Current, W. L., Rose, N. C., Ernst, J. V., Bailey, W., Heyman, M., and Weinstein, W. (1983). Human cryptosporidiosis in immunocompetent and immunodeficient persons–Studies of an outbreak and experimental transmission. *N. Engl. J. Med.* **308**:1252-1257.

Davidson, P. T. (1982). Treatment of infections due to atypical mycobacteria. In *Current Clinical Topics in Infectious Diseases,* vol. III.

DeJong, J., Valderrama, G., Spigland, I., and Horowitz, M. S. (1983). Adenovirus isolates from urine of patients with acquired immunodeficiency syndrome. *Lancet* **1**:1293-1296.

Drew, W. L., Mintz, L., Miner, R. C., Sands, M., and Ketterer, B. (1981). Prevalence of cytomegalovirus infection in homosexual men. *J. Infect. Dis.* **143**:188-192.

Dutt, A., and Stead, W. W. (1979). Long term results of medical treatment in Mycobacterium intracellulare infection. *Am. J. Med.* **67**:449-453.

Elliott, J., Hoppes, W., Platt, M. S., Thomas, J. G., Patel, I. P., and Gansar, A. (1983). The acquired immunodeficiency syndrome and Mycobacterium avium-intracellulare bacteremia in a patient with hemophilia. *Ann. Int. Med.* **98**:290-293.

Fainstein, V., Bolivar, R., Mavligit, G., Rios A., and Luna, M. (1982). Disseminated infection due to Mycobacterium avium-intracellulare in a homosexual man with Kaposi's sarcoma. *J. Infect. Dis.* **145**:586.

Follansbee, S. E., Busch, D. F., Wofsy, C. B., Coleman, D. L., Gullet, J., Aurigemma, G. P., Ross, T., Hadley, W. V., and Drew, W. L. (1982). An outbreak of *Pneumocystis carinii* pneumonia in homosexual men. *Ann. Int. Med.* **96**:705-713.

Friedman-Kien, A. E., Laubenstein, L. J., Rubinstein, P., Buimovici-Klein, E., Marmor, M., Stahl, R., Spigland, I., Kim, K. S., and Zolla-Pazner, S. (1982). Disseminated Kaposi's sarcoma in homosexual men. *Ann. Int. Med.* **96**:693-700.

Gamsu, G., Hecht, S. T., Birnberg, F. A. Coleman, D. L., and Golden, J. A. (1982). *Pneumocystis carinii* in homosexual men. *Am. J. Roentgenol.* **139**:647-651.

Golden, J. (1982). Pneumocystis lung disease in homosexual men–Medical Staff Conference, University of California, San Francisco. *West. J. Med.* **137**:400-407.

Gottlieb, M., Schroff, R., Schanker, H. M., Weisman, J. D., Fan, P. T., Wolf, R. A., and Saxon, A. (1981). *Pneumocystis carinii* pneumonia and mucosal candidiasis in previously healthy homosexual men–evidence of a new acquired cellular immunodeficiency. *N. Engl. J. Med.* **305**:1425-1431.

Gottlieb, M. S., Groopman, J. E., Weinstein, W. M., Fahey, J. L., and Detels, R. (1983). The acquired immunodeficiency syndrome. *Ann. Int. Med.* **99**:208-220.

Greene, J., Sidhu, G., Lewin, S., Levine, J. F., Masur, H., Simberkoff, M. S., Nicholas, P., Good, R. C., Zolla-Pazner, S., Pollock, A., Tapper, M. L., and Holzman, R. S. (1982). Mycobacterium avium-intracellulare: A cause of disseminated life-threatening infection in homosexuals and drug abusers. *Ann. Int. Med.* **97**:539-546.

Ho, M. (1982). *Cytomegalovirus—Biology and Infection.* New York, Plenum Press.

Holland, G. N., Gottlieb, M. S., Yee, R. D., Schanker, H. M., and Petit, T. H. (1982). Ocular disorders associated with a new severe acquired cellular immunodeficiency syndrome. *Am. J. Ophthalmol.* **93**:393-402.

Horowitz, S. L., Bentson, J. R., Benson, D. F., Davos, I., Pressman, B., and Gottlieb, M. S. (1983). Toxoplasmosis in a new acquired cellular immunodeficiency syndrome. *Arch. Neurol.* **40**:649-652.

Hughes, W. T., Kuhn, S., Chaudhary, S., Feldman, S., Verzosa, M., Aur, R. J. A., Pratt, C., and George, S. L. (1977). Successful chemoprophylaxis for *Pneumocystis carinii* pneumonitis. *N. Engl. J. Med.* **297**: 1419-1426.

Hughes, W. T. (1979). Limited effect of trimethoprim-sulfamethoxazole prophylaxis on *Pneumocystis carinii. Antimicrob. Agents Chemother.* **16**: 333-335.

Hughes, W. T., Bartley, D. L., and Smith, B. M. (1983). A natural source of infection due to *Pneumocystis carinii. J. Infect. Dis.* **147**:595.

Jaffe, H., Choi, K., Thomas, P. A., Haverkos, H. W., Auerbach, D. M., Guinan, M. E., Rogers, M. F., Spira, T. J., Darrow, W. W., Kramer, M. A., Friedman, S. M., Monroe, J. M., Safai, B., Dritz, S. K., Crispi, S. J., Fanin, S. L., Orkwis, J. P., Kelter, A., Rushing, W. R., Thacker, S. B., and Curran, J. W. (1983). National case-control study of Kaposi's sarcoma and *Pneumocystis carinii* pneumonia in homosexual men: Part I, Epidemiologic results. *Ann. Int. Med.* **99**:145-151.

Kluge, R. M., Spaulding, D. M., and Spain, J. A. (1978). Combination of pentamidine and trimethoprim-sulfamethoxazole in the therapy of *Pneumocystis carinii* pneumonia in rat. *Antimicrob. Agents Chemotherap.* **13**:975-978.

Ma, P., and Soave, R. (1983). Three-step stool examination for Cryptosporidiosis in 10 homosexual men with protracted watery diarrhea. *J. Infect. Dis.* **147**:824-828.

Masur, M., Michelis, M. A., Greene, J. B., Onarato, I., Stouwe, R. A. V., Holzman, R. S., Wormser, G., Brettman, L., Lange, M., Murray, H. W., and Cunningham-Rundles, S. (1981). An outbreak of community-acquired *Pneumocystis carinii* pneumonia–Initial manifestations of cellular immune dysfunction. *N. Engl. J. Med.* **305**:1431-1438.

Masur, H., Michelis, M. A., Wormser, G. P., Lewin, S., Gold, J., Tapper, M. L., Giron, J., Lerner, C. W., Armstrong, D., Setia, V., Sender, J. A., Seilkin, R. S., Nicholas, P., Arlen, Z., Maayan, S., Maayan, S., Ernst, J. A., Siegel, F. B., and Cunningham-Rundles, S. (1982). Opportunistic infection in previously healthy women–Initial manifestations of a community-acquired cellular immunodeficiency. *Ann. Int. Med.* **97**:533-539.

McCauley, D. I., Naidich, D. P., Leitman, N. S., Reede, D. L., and Laubenstein, L. (1982). Radiographic patterns of opportunistic lung infections and Kaposi sarcoma in homosexual men. *Am. J. Roentgenol.* **139**:653-658.

Menitore, J. E., Aster, R. H., Casper, J. T., Lauer, S. J., Gottschall, J. L., Williams, J. E., Gill, J. C., Wheeler, D. V., Piaskowski, V., Kirchner, P., and Montgomery, R. R. (1983). T lymphocyte subpopulations in patients with classic hemophilia treated with cryoprecipitate and lyophilized concentrates. *N. Engl. J. Med.* **308**:83-86.

Meyers, J. D., and Thomas, E. D. (1981). Infection Complicating Bone Marrow Transplantation. In *Clinical Approach to Infection in the Compromised Host.* Edited by R. Rubin and L. Young. New York, Plenum Publishing, pp. 507-551.

Mildvan, D., Mathur, V., Enlow, R. W., Romain, P. L., Winchester, R. J., Culp, C., Singman, H., Adelsberg, B. R., and Spigland, I. (1982). Opportunistic infections and immune deficiency in homosexual men. *Ann. Int. Med.* **96**:700-704.

Miller, J. R., Barrett, R. E., Britton, C. B., Tapper, M. L., Bahr, G. S., Bruno, P. J., Marquardt, M. D., Hays, A. P., McMurtry, J. G., Weissman, J. B., and Bruno, M. S. (1982). Progressive multifocal leukoencephalopathy in a male homosexual with T-cell immune deficiency. *N. Engl. J. Med.* **307**:1436-1438.

Mitsuyasu, R., Groopman, J., and Volberding, P. (1983). Reaction to trimethoprim-sulfamethoxazole in patients with AIDS and Kaposi's sarcoma. *N. Engl. J. Med.* **308**:1535.

Neuwirth, J., Gutman, I., Hofeldt, A., Behrens, M., Marquardt, M. D., Abramovsky-Kaplan, I., Kelsey, P., and Odel, J. (1982). Cytomegalovirus retinitis in a young homosexual male with acquired immunodeficiency. *Ophthalmology* **89**:805-808.

Pitchenik, A. E., Fischl, M. A., and Wall, K. W. (1983a). Evaluation of cerebral-mass lesions in acquired immunodeficiency syndrome. *N. Engl. J. Med.* **308**:1099.

Pitchenik, A., Fischl, M. A., Dickinson, G. M., Becker, D. M., Fournier, A. M., O'Connell, M. T., Colton, R. M., and Spira, T. J. (1983b). Opportunistic infections and Kaposi's sarcoma among Haitians: Evidence of a new acquired immunodeficiency state. *Ann. Int. Med.* **98**:277-284.

Poon, M., Lauday, A., Prasthofer, E. F., and Stagno, S. (1983). Acquired immunodeficiency syndrome with *Pneumocystis carinii* pneumonia and Mycobacterium avium-intracellular infection in a previously healthy patient with classic hemophilia—clinical, immunologic and virologic findings. *Ann. Int. Med.* **98**:287-290.

Rogers, M. F., Morens, D. M., Stewart, J. A., Kaminski, R. M., Spira, T. J., Feorino, P. M., Larsen, S. A., Francis, D. P., Wilson, M., and Kaufman, L. (1983). National case-control study of Kaposi's sarcoma and *Pneumocystis carinii* pneumonia in homosexual men. Part 2. Laboratory results. *Ann. Int. Med.* **99**:151-158.

Ruskin, J. (1981). Parasitic Disease in the Compromised Host. In *Clinical Approach to Infection in the Compromised Host.* Edited by R. Rubin and L. Young. New York, Plenum Publishing, pp. 311-323.

Sattler, F. R., and Remington, J. S. (1981). Intravenous trimethoprim-sulfamethoxazole therapy for *Pneumocystis carinii* pneumonia. *Am. J. Med.* **70**:1215-1221.

Siegal, F. P., Lopez, C., Hammer, G. S., Brown, A. E., Kornfeld, S. J., Gold, J., Hassett, J., Hirschman, S. Z., Cunningham-Rundles, C., Adelsberg, B. R., Parham, D., Siegel, M., Cunningham-Rundles, S., and Armstrong, D. (1981). Severe acquired immunodeficiency in male homosexuals, manifested by chronic perianal ulcertive herpes simplex lesions. *N. Engl. J. Med.* **305**:1439-1444.

Small, C. B., Klein, R. S., Friedland, G. H., Moll, B., Emeson, E. E., and Spigland, I. (1983). Community-acquired opportunistic infections and defective cellular immunity in heterosexual drug abusers and homosexual men. *Am. J. Med.* **74**:433-441.

Tzipori, S. (1983). Cryptosporidiosis in animals and humans. *Microbiol. Rev.* **47**:84-96.

Vanley, G., Huberman, R., and Lufkin, R. (1982). Atypical *Pneumocystis carinii* pneumonia in homosexual men with unusual immunodeficiency. *Am. J. Roentgenol.* **138**:1037-1041.

Vieira, J., Frank, E., Spira, T., and Landesman, S. H. (1983). Acquired immune deficiency in Haitians—Opportunistic infections in previously healthy Haitian immigrants. *N. Engl. J. Med.* **308**:125-129.

Walzer, P. D., Perl, D. P., Krogstad, D. J., Rawson, P. G., and Schultz, M. G. (1974). *Pneumocystis carinii* pneumonia in the United States—Epidemiologic, diagnostic and clinical features. *Ann. Int. Med.* **80**:83-93.

Westerman, E. L., and Christensen, R. P. (1979). Chronic Isospora belli infection treated with Cotrimoxazole. *Ann. Int. Med.* **91**:413-414.

Winston, D. J., Lau, W. K., Gale, R. P., and Young, L. S. (1980). Trimethoprim-sulfamethoxazole for the treatment of *Pneumocystis carinii* pneumonia. *Ann. Int. Med.* **92**:762-769.

Wolinsky, E. (1979). Nontuberculous mycobacteria and associated diseases. *Am. Rev. Resp. Dis.* **119**:107-159.

Wormser, G. P., Krupp, L. B., Hanrahan, J. P., Gavis, G., Spira, T. J., and Cunningham-Rundles, S. (1983). Acquired immunodeficiency syndrome in male prisoners—new insights into an emerging syndrome. *Ann. Int. Med.* **98**:197-303.

Young, L. S. (1982). Trimethoprim-sulfamethoxazole in the treatment of adults with pneumonia due to *Pneumocystis carinii. Rev. Infect. Dis.* **4**:608-613.

Zakowski, P., Fligiel S., Berlin, O. G., and Johnson, B. L. (1982). Disseminated Mycobacterium avium-intracellulare. Infection in homosexual men dying of acquired immunodeficiency. *JAMA* **248**:2980-2982.

AUTHOR INDEX

Italic numbers give the page on which the complete reference is listed.

Y

Z

SUBJECT INDEX

A

Acquired immunodeficiency syndrome (AIDS)
definition of, 195-196
guidelines for care of patients with, 219
major clinical findings in, 197-200
other opportunistic infections and, 212-220
Pneumocystis carinii pneumonia and, 207-212
Actinomycin D, 206

B

Bacterial infections, AIDS and, 213
Bleomycin, 147
Bronchoalveolar lavage, 164
Burkitt's lymphoma, 205

C

Candida albicans, 145
Candida pseudotropicalis, 108
Chest pain, 149
Clinical aspects of pneumocystosis in man, 139-174
clinical manifestations of infection, 147-151

[Clinical aspects of pneumocystosis in man]
diagnostic approaches, 154-168
approach to diagnosis and management, 165-167
dilemma of nonspecific or negative lung biopsy, 167-168
pros and cons of establishing diagnosis, 159-165
radiologic manifestations, 156-159
epidemiology, 139-147
data on incidence and underlying disease, 142-144
outbreak in patients with apparent acquired immunodeficiency, 144-147
laboratory findings, 151-154
sequelae, 168
Clinical manifestations of pneumocystis infection, 147-151
Coccidioisis, 215
Concanavalin A, 145
Corticosteroids, acute reinstitution of, 186
Coughing, 148, 149, 150
Cryptococcus neoformans, 145
Cryptosporidia, 145
Cryptosporidium, 214-215
Cultivation, 3
Cutting needle biopsy, 164
Cytomegalovirus (CMV), 145, 201, 205-206, 217-218